Second Edition

ENDING
NURSE-TO-NURSE
HOSTILITY

Why Nurses Eat Their
Young and Each Other

Kathleen Bartholomew, RN, MN

Kathleen Bartholomew, RN, MN, Author
Rebecca Hendren, Product Manager
Mary-Anne Benedict, MSN, RN, Lead Nurse Planner
Elizabeth Petersen, Vice President
Vincent Skyers, Design Manager
Michael McCalip, Layout/Graphic Design

Claudette Moore, Acquisitions Editor
Erin Callahan, Senior Director, Product
Kerry Neenan, Continuing Education Manager
Matt Sharpe, Production Supervisor
Vicki McMahan, Sr. Graphic Designer
Kelly Church, Cover Designer

Contents

To access the sample tools and documents included in this book, visit the link below.

www.hcpro.com/downloads/11641

Dedication

With great admiration and love to all the Orthopedic and Spine staff of the Swedish Orthopedic Institute in Seattle—the wind beneath my wings.

Acknowledgements

To the numerous researchers who have dedicated their energy and time to understanding our relationships with each other, most notably Sandra Thomas, RN, PhD, FAAN, Gerald Farrell, RN, PhD, Martha Griffin, PhD, RN, CNS, FAAN, and Cynthia Clark, PhD, RN, ANEF, FAAN; my teachers, Genevieve Bartol, RN, EdD, AHN-C(P), and Linda Westbrook, RN, PhD; colleagues, Brady G. Wilson (Juice, Inc.), Deb Cox and Dianne Jacobs (CoMass), John Nelson, PhD, MS, RN; AnnMarie Papa, RN, FAAN; and my ever-patient and supportive husband, John Nance.

About the Author

Kathleen Bartholomew, RN, MN

Before turning to healthcare as a career in 1994, Kathleen Bartholomew held positions in marketing, business, communications, and teaching. It was these experiences that allowed her to look at the culture of healthcare from a unique perspective and speak poignantly to the issues affecting providers and the challenges facing organizations today.

Bartholomew has been a national speaker since 2001. As the manager of a large surgical unit in Seattle, she quickly recognized that creating a culture where staff felt a sense of belonging was critical to retention. During her tenure as manager, staff, physician, and patient satisfaction reached the top 10% as she implemented her down-to-earth strategies. Despite the nursing shortage, she could always depend on a waiting list of nurses for both units.

Her bachelor's degree is in liberal arts with a strong emphasis on sociology. This background laid the foundation for her to correctly identify the norms particular to healthcare—specifically physician-nurse relationships and nurse-to-nurse hostility. For her master's thesis, she authored *Speak Your Truth: Proven Strategies for Effective Nurse-Physician Communication,* the only book to date which addresses physician-nurse issues.

In December of 2005, Bartholomew resigned her position as manager in order to write the first edition of *Ending Nurse-to-Nurse Hostility*, her second book on horizontal violence in nursing. The expression "nurses eat their young" has existed for many years in the nursing profession (and has troubled many in the profession). Her book offered the first comprehensive and compassionate look at the etiology, impact, and solutions to horizontal violence. She won the best media depiction of nursing for her op editorial in *The Seattle Post Intelligencer* and in 2010 she was nominated by HealthLeaders Media as one of the top 20 people changing healthcare in America.

Bartholomew's passion for creating healthy work environments is infectious. She is an expert on hospital culture and speaks internationally to hospital boards, the military, leadership, and staff about safety, communication, cultural change, and power. With her husband, John J. Nance, she co-authored *Charting the Course: Launching Patient-Centric Healthcare* in 2012, which is the sequel to *Why Hospitals Should Fly* (2008).

From the bedside to the boardroom, Kathleen Bartholomew applies research to practice with humor and an ethical call to excellence that ignites and inspires health caregivers and leaders to unprecedented levels of excellence.

Other books authored or coauthored by Kathleen Bartholomew, RN, MN

Speak Your Truth

Stressed Out About Communication Skills

Charting the Course

Educational video and audio (Information at *www.kathleenbartholomew.com*)

Ending Nurse-to-Nurse Hostility: Raising Awareness

Ending Nurse-to-Nurse Hostility: Powerful Conversations

Creating Healthy Relationships (CEUs: 4)

Nursing Continuing Education

For information on earning 4 hours of Continuing Nursing Education credits, and to download additional materials supporting this book, visit your downloads page: *www.hcpro.com/downloads/11641*.

Learning objectives for *Ending Nurse-to-Nurse Hostility,* Second Edition:

1. Define horizontal hostility.
2. List two overt examples of horizontal hostility from your work setting.
3. List two covert examples of horizontal hostility from your work setting.
4. Discuss the impact that horizontal hostility has on 1) the individual and 2) the organization.
5. Explain the impact that horizontal hostility has on patient safety.
6. Explain one way in which the current system is designed to support the invisibility of nurses.
7. List two populations at risk for experiencing horizontal hostility.
8. State four of the most frequent forms of lateral violence.
9. Explain why horizontal hostility is so virulent.
10. Identify two intrinsic forces that play a role in horizontal hostility.
11. Explain how the organizational structure enables oppression.
12. Select two factors that contribute to nurses' stress from the context of our world.
13. List two impediments to a healthy student or resident nurse experience.
14. Describe six steps that can be taken to create a healthy environment for student nurses.
15. Name two signs that may indicate that horizontal hostility is taking place.
16. Explain what is meant by a "twofold approach" to eliminating horizontal hostility.
17. Select one way in which nurse managers can empower staff.
18. Identify two strategies to nurture a healthy culture within the organization.
19. Identify two strategies to decrease hostility within the organization.
20. Identify two practices or behaviors characteristic of an open system.

Prologue

Skye is a nursing assistant on our unit. Despite having a bachelor's degree in public health and a 3.9 GPA, she is still number 54 on a waiting list for nursing school. Her goal is to gain experience by working as a nursing assistant and eventually become a nursing instructor. However, the experience she is gaining at our hospital isn't just limited to clinical practice.

On this particular morning, she and I are watching the drama unfold as the charge nurses argue over staffing for the floor. There is no point in intervening. It is just a few minutes before 7 a.m., and I have counseled both nurses in the past. Emotions are high, and the nurses are arriving at good decisions for the floor despite their arguments.

Finally, everyone goes into report and Skye looks at me with a puzzled expression. "Why the drama?" she asks. I remember that yesterday Skye worked with two staff nurses who spent the entire shift venting about one another—to everyone on the floor but each other. "Is this what they mean by nurses eating their young and each other?" she asks hesitantly.

I take a deep breath. Horizontal hostility is a complex problem with many facets, and I don't want to gloss it over or turn her off to nursing. I want Skye to truly see and understand the forces that create and maintain this problem. It would be just as much of a disservice to Skye as it would be to nursing not to answer this question thoroughly and honestly. Drawing upon my own experience as a nurse manager, as well as research that has been conducted in the United States and other countries, I turn my answer into a book.

Section 1

Understanding the Forces

Chapter 1

What Is Horizontal Hostility?

Define your terms, and I will speak with you.

—*Voltaire*

Defining Horizontal Hostility

When I began researching horizontal violence in 2005, there were approximately 200 articles in PubMed with the vast majority listed under "verbal abuse." Today, there are thousands of peer-reviewed papers, and a Google search will yield more than 600,000 hits. But after almost a decade of research, there are still numerous terms used to describe these negative interactions among humans:

- Interactive workplace trauma, anger, relational aggression, horizontal hostility, bullying, incivility, verbal abuse, and horizontal or lateral violence.

These terms are then further subdivided within relationships: nurse-to-doctor, patient-to-nurse, and nurse-to-nurse. Researchers agree that all of these terms fall into the category of **disruptive behavior,** which may be defined as:

> *... any behavior that interferes with effective communication among healthcare providers and negatively impacts performance and outcomes.*
>
> —*Center for American Nurses Position Statement*

Although the literature provides a better understanding of the presence and effect of negative emotions in healthcare settings, the lack of a single universal term makes it quite a challenge to integrate the research into one cohesive picture or to study the prevalence. The following are just some of the definitions used in literature on the subject:

♦ **Incivility:** "Rude or disruptive behaviors which often result in psychological or physiological distress for the people involved—and if left unaddressed, may progress to threatening situations" (Clark, 2013).

♦ **Verbal abuse:** "Communication perceived by a person to be a harsh, condemnatory attack, either professional or personal. Language intended to cause distress to a target" (Buback, 2004).

♦ **Bullying:** "The persistent, demeaning, and downgrading of humans through vicious words and cruel acts that gradually undermine confidence and self-esteem" (Adams, 1997).

Initial research on aggression in nursing came from Australia and Great Britain, where bullying is a much broader term which includes aggression from superiors, subordinates, and peers in the workplace. The definition of bullying shares three elements that come from racial and sexual harassment law. "First, bullying is defined in terms of its effect on the recipient—not the intention of the bully. Secondly, there must be a negative effect on the victim. Thirdly, the bullying behavior must be persistent" (Quine, 1999).

In America, however, the term "bullying" is most commonly used to refer to someone who holds power over you whether formally or informally. For example, a charge nurse has the power over the assignment and can use that power to punish a nurse by giving him or her a bad assignment—or a manager can bully by refusing a vacation request for no apparent reason other than retaliation because the nurse called in sick a week earlier.

◆ **Horizontal violence:** "Sabotage directed at coworkers who are on the same level within an organization's hierarchy" (Dunn, 2003).

◆ **Horizontal hostility**: "A consistent pattern of behavior designed to control, diminish, or devalue a peer (or group) that creates a risk to health and/or safety" (Farrell, 2005).

The terms "horizontal hostility" and "lateral violence" are used to portray aggressive behavior between individuals on the same power level, such as nurse-to-nurse and manager-to-manager. Because "violence" infers physical acts of aggression for many people, I use the term "horizontal hostility," as defined by Gerald Farrell, RN, PhD, and congruent with the elements of harassment law listed above. Ironically, researchers have found that the more indirect, covert incivilities (like denigration) resulted in more extensive emotional trauma and stress than did outright physical abuse (Mayhew et al., 2004).

Overt and covert behavior—Call it what it is!

A Chinese magician's apprentice asked, "Master, how do you take the power away from something?" "That's easy," replied his master. "You just call it by its name."

Horizontal hostility can be either overt or covert. It can also take many forms: physical, verbal, nonverbal, or psychological. The psychological forms of hostility are often covert, which makes the behaviors a challenge for managers to address. A lack of cooperation, poor teamwork, refusing to help someone or pretending you are too busy, blaming, and withholding information are all forms of psychological hostility (Blair, 2013).

Since studies show that the majority of our communication is nonverbal, and stress is heightened in ambiguous situations, covert behaviors have the biggest impact.

◆ **Overt:** Name-calling, bickering, fault-finding, backstabbing, criticism, intimidation, gossip, shouting, blaming, using put-downs, raising eyebrows, eye-rolling (perceived), ignoring someone's greeting, nicknames, failing to give credit when due, etc.

- ◆ **Covert:** Unfair assignments, sarcasm, eye-rolling (behind someone's back), ignoring, making faces behind someone's back, refusing to help, sighing, whining, refusing to work with someone, sabotage, isolation, exclusion, fabrication, etc.

Examples of these covert and overt behaviors run as a continuous thread through the numerous stories I have heard throughout my career. I have incorporated these stories into this book. The following is an example of overt hostility experienced by a fellow nurse:

I am used to being in a charge nurse position and am now working with recovering patients from the cath lab. The hostility here is thinly veiled. I come into work and say something like, "Nice day today," and the charge replies, "What's that supposed to mean?"

We have really sick patients just fresh out of the cath lab. When the charge nurse told me she was going to take a break, I asked her a few questions so I would have the information I needed to cover. I asked, "Does 212 have a sheath in?" and the charge nurse said, "What do you want to know for?" I try to ignore her and just do my job.

When she came back from break I told her all that had happened in her absence— for example, that I taped down the IV in 214. Coldly, she responded, "That could've waited until I returned."

It's a constant, negative, put-you-down undercurrent that never ends.

Continuum of harm

Dr. Cindy Clark recognized that hostile and rude behaviors occur on a wide spectrum of harm that ranges from low to high risk and from disruptive to threatening. Her work gives perspective to negative acts and helps leaders to understand that if left unaddressed, hostile behaviors can escalate. For example, eye-rolling and sarcastic comments would be classified as low risk and intimidation and physical violence as high risk (Clark, 2013).

Figure 1.1   The wide spectrum of harm from hostile behaviors

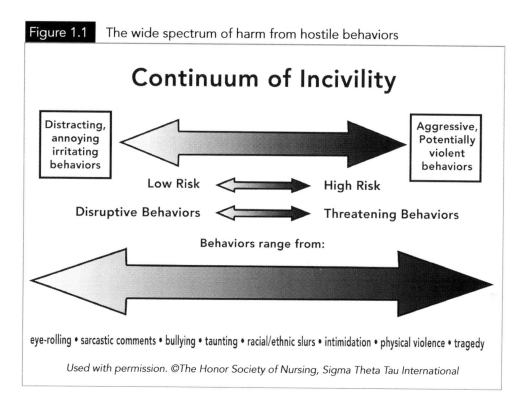

Continuum of Incivility

Distracting, annoying irritating behaviors ⟵⟶ Aggressive, Potentially violent behaviors

Low Risk ⟷ High Risk

Disruptive Behaviors ⟷ Threatening Behaviors

Behaviors range from:

eye-rolling • sarcastic comments • bullying • taunting • racial/ethnic slurs • intimidation • physical violence • tragedy

Used with permission. ©The Honor Society of Nursing, Sigma Theta Tau International

In June 2010, after the death of an operating room nurse, the government in Ontario passed "Bully Busting Bill 168" in order to raise awareness of the critical need to address low-risk, disruptive behaviors that, if left ignored, can result in tragedy. This bill is an amendment to the Occupational Health and Safety Act and requires organizations to develop a policy, educate employees, post the policy, and conduct a risk assessment. Bystanders who witness harassment now have a moral, ethical, and legal obligation to act. Examples of harassment include making remarks, jokes, or innuendos that demean, ridicule, intimidate, or offend. The OSHA definition is:

◆   **Workplace harassment**: "Engaging in a course of vexatious comment or conduct against a worker in a workplace that is known or ought reasonably to be known to be unwelcome." Any repeated words or actions, or a pattern of behaviors, against a worker or group of workers in the workplace that are unwelcome are considered harassment.

Is Horizontal Hostility Intentional?

For more than an hour, Bethany has been recounting examples of horizontal hostility over a 14-year career, which brought her to three different states and through major depression. At the end of the interview, I ask her, "Do you think the nurses knew what they were doing? Were their actions intentional?"

She bristles and responds almost indignantly, "Their actions were very intentional. They knew exactly what they were doing!"

I press further, "But were their actions conscious? Do you think those nurses were aware of the pain they were causing you?"

Bethany pauses and her face softens. "No, they were clueless to the effect of their actions. They never looked past [their actions] to see how another person would feel. What got me was how a person could hate someone they didn't even know."

The above scenario has occurred with hundreds of nurses whom I have counseled. The intent of backstabbing, intimidation, fault-finding, etc., is to alienate, attack, or punish a coworker. However, in the majority of cases, the perpetrators did not understand the consequences of their actions. Many believed that they were superior because they were upholding a particular standard of quality patient care.

Only through education, which began by raising awareness of the damage and confronting the behavior, did nurses begin to comprehend the full extent of their actions. And when a nurse did "get it," the behavior stopped immediately. This is the reason horizontal hostility is such a threat to our profession: because it is so insidious. Nurses do not perceive the harm that they are causing. And the harm is devastating.

Victims are as wounded as if the attack had been physical. They suffer for months, fear more abuse, function apprehensively, and believe that there is something wrong with them—that they are not good enough or "not cut out to be a nurse."

In a study of 227 nurses, over one-third of nurses admitted that they had engaged in negative behaviors. When nurses were asked to reflect on why, they said they were "sadly caught up in the moment" and expressed disappointment in themselves for participating in the negativity (Walrafen et al., 2012).

Opportunity: Understanding how humans behave in groups

The greatest need of the soul is for belonging.

—*Thomas Moore*

We have both an opportunity and an obligation to listen to nurses' stories and learn from these experiences in order to create a new reality: a healthy workplace for each other and our patients. We can start by learning more about human behavior in groups.

When humans become part of a new group, they adopt the behaviors of that group in order to be accepted because the threat of exclusion is so devastating. This process— where we unconsciously accept the behaviors of the group—is called assimilation. For example, if you join a unit and hear nurses constantly talking and gossiping about someone, then before long you will find yourself doing the same thing. While you may have been surprised at the gossiping at first, the behavior becomes normal because no one ever challenges it, and you see frequent examples every day (Ceravolo et al., 2012).

Not only do staff members match the behavior of each other, but they also normalize behaviors and tolerate a culture of hostility when the supervisor is the source of the abuse (Hutchinson et al., 2010). The collective belief established appeared to be, *"If the manager can behave that way, then everyone else can too."*

In short, the more people that watch a behavior, the less chance that someone will actually intervene. Responsibility diffuses in a crowd.

Opportunity: Understanding powerful emotions

The expression "nurses eat their young" has existed for as long as nurses can remember. We secretly acknowledge the culture to each other, yet never admit this out loud. This aphorism implies that there is a problem specifically within the nursing profession and is accompanied by a feeling of shame. This is the primary reason why it has taken us so long to address the issue. But the more I researched the phenomena of horizontal hostility, the more I realized that I was studying all human behavior— not just nursing behavior.

In her pivotal book, *Odd Girl Out,* Rachel Simmons zeroes in on the hidden culture of aggression in teenagers. She points out these very same overt and covert behaviors happening between middle school students. Or perhaps you remember your high school cliques? In that setting, gossip was used to spread information on how each person was supposed to behave (so that the person listening learned how not to behave). The person who spread the gossip gained power and status because they had the "goods"—or the information—that no one else had (Brooks, 2011).

> *We tell ourselves stories about those who violate the rules of our group both to reinforce our connections with one another and to remind ourselves of the standards that bind us together.*
>
> —Haidt, The Righteous Mind

It is difficult to admit that we could be hurting each other in a profession that has its fundamental roots in caring. Uncovering and discussing horizontal hostility is about as easy as a family acknowledging how damaging it is to live with alcoholism. It is embarrassing and is so remotely removed from our idea of the perfect nurse that we shudder to think that it may be true.

In addition, there is an unspoken fear, warranted or not, that acknowledging the problem will make it worse. However, if nursing is to survive, we need an immediate intervention. This intervention starts with listening to the voices in the room—the researchers who have uncovered this behavior, and the nurses who are experiencing the hostility.

Tales From the Front Line

> *Our communication is fraught with indirect aggression, bickering, and fault-finding. It is disheartening to experience the underhanded and devastating ways that nurses attack each other. These rifts divide us and lead us to injure one another.*
>
> —Laura Gasparis Vonfrolio, RN, PhD

There is nothing as powerful as a story. Stories put the truth out into the world—once a story is shared, you cannot call it back. Stories are a means of truth-telling. If we have had a similar experience, a story resonates with us at the deepest level, and there is comfort and validation as we realize that others share our experience.

At the "Horizontal Violence in the Workplace" conference held by the Oregon chapter of the American Psychiatric Nurses Association, I asked participants whether they would be willing to share their stories about hostility in the workplace. I collected a list of names and phone numbers of interested nurses and arranged convenient times to speak to each one by phone. As I listened to the first story, I was shocked at the intensity of aggression the nurse had experienced and by the fact that the continual verbal abuse had resulted in a suicide attempt.

From hospitals and academia to outpatient clinic settings, nurses shared with me their poignant experiences with horizontal hostility. Research shows that these stories are not isolated events and that the effects of these negative emotions have a serious impact. "Horizontal hostility drains nurses of vitality and undermines institutional attempts to create a satisfied nursing workforce" (Thomas, 2003).

> *This is what the group of nurses would do to me: I never sat down for 12 hours. It was horrendous. All I know is that if a group works together for long enough, they keep the others outside.*

> *The smallest thing would trigger retaliation. [The charge nurse's] refusal to speak was the worst. Once she went 27 days without speaking.*

> *It was the looks [the preceptor] gave me, like I was stupid. In my whole three months of orientation, I can't think of a single time anyone ever complimented me.*

> *The orientation nurse was ultimately fired. She started drinking and felt attacked all the time. Everything was her fault, all the time.*

As nurses shared their experiences with me, two common themes emerged. First, every single participant was gravely concerned about maintaining anonymity for fear of being identified. Even if the violence had happened 10 years ago and had been resolved by the abuser leaving the workplace, all nurses feared retaliation. The workplace was still viewed as dangerous, and nurses continued to feel vulnerable.

Secondly, no matter what the situation, the stories clearly brought up a lot of emotional pain that was difficult to acknowledge. Like those suffering from post traumatic stress disorder, participants appeared to be reliving their hurt all over again.

The air was still thick with feelings of loss and betrayal after the conversations were finished. As stories were coaxed from each nurse, the courage required to tell their stories became obvious. Even to be a witness to another's story was upsetting:

> Survivors have to look the other way ... or go along with the crowd to survive.
> You have to take the party line even if you don't believe it.

When asked to reflect on horizontal hostility, people can frequently identify the bully but fail to realize the critical importance of the supporting roles. Witnesses reported feeling two types of anger: a generally angry mood and a personally targeted anger toward the offender (Porath, 2009).

The "silent witness" is a term used to identify people who watch the behavior but say or do nothing. By their apathy and silence, witnesses allow the practice of bullying to continue as an acceptable norm. Because responsibility diffuses in a crowd, witnesses frequently do not feel the need to act. Also, many witnesses report feeling relieved that the bullying or hostility is not directed at them. Many report that their biggest fear is that by speaking up and becoming visible, they will inadvertently redirect the hostility toward themselves.

The target or victim is another key player in the horizontal hostility drama. As we will discuss in later chapters, the most vulnerable target is always someone who is different from the group. Targets are not limited to the new nurse—now there are several reports of older nurses being targeted with hostile behaviors. The only criteria is being different. Therefore, the manager who reaches unprecedented levels of patient or employee satisfaction can also be a target.

The unspoken and unconscious motive of the hostility is homogeneity. Powerless groups travel like a school of fish in order to stay psychologically safe.

Horizontal hostility exists at all levels

> I was standing next to the executive director for recruitment and retention for a West Coast state. I was thrilled because I had just been invited on to a radio program in San Francisco that would reach over a million listeners. But when I shared this information with her, she immediately responded, "That shouldn't be you—it should be a California nurse. Why do you get to go?"

I was the outgoing president of a nursing organization representing over 20,000 nurses. During her acceptance speech the new president announced, "And I want you to know that THIS year we will be doing things right!" I sat in the audience mortified as several peers emailed their disbelief and sympathies at the words they were hearing.

A lead instructor of mine rolls her eyes and huffs when asked a question ... she makes all of us feel as if we are wasting her time, and begins every class by saying, "We have a lot to cover today so don't ask any questions."

I was supposed to have two faculty mentors for my graduate project. But they refused to talk to each other, or meet me together ... and so I felt like a Ping-Pong ball and wasted a tremendous amount of time redoing work.

From staff nurse to chief nursing officer, nurses have reported experiencing hostile behaviors. No one is exempt. To be dissed by the profession that you have dedicated your life to is simply devastating. Frequently, however, nurses minimize the impact because they internalize the pain. They believe these situations only happen to them because they don't know how frequently these behaviors occur elsewhere.

Prevalence in the U.S. and Beyond

How frequently do these behaviors actually occur? The larger body of literature reflects a huge spread of incidence of horizontal hostility, experienced by as few as 18% to a high of 76% of those surveyed (Vessey et al., 2011). One reason for this wide spread is because hostility was defined and measured differently across the various studies by different researchers. The most consistent information about prevalence came from two rigorous studies that used the same reliable and valid measures. These two studies found a prevalence rate of 27% and 31% respectively of nurses who experienced hostility (Purpora et al., 2012).

Horizontal hostility in nursing is not unique to the United States. On an international level, one in three nurses plans to leave his or her position because of horizontal hostility (McMillan, 1995). In 1996, a survey was conducted of more than 1,100 employees of a National Health Service Community Trust in England, which included 396 nurses. The bullied staff reported lower job satisfaction, higher job stress, greater depression and anxiety, and greater intent to leave their job. The bully was a superior in 54% of cases, a peer in 34%, and a subordinate 12% of the time. Thirty percent of respondents in the study stated that they were subjected to aggression "on a daily or near daily basis" (Farrell, 1999).

A study in the United Kingdom of 4,500 nurses showed that one in six nurses reported that they had experienced workplace mistreatment in the past year and that 33% were intending to leave the workplace because of verbal abuse. Mistreatment by peers accounted for 41% of verbal abuse (Gilmour and Hamlin, 2003).

Studies in the United States indicate that 90%–97% of nurses experience verbal abuse from physicians (Manderino and Berkey, 1997). Some speculate that verbal abuse by physicians contributes significantly to horizontal hostility because nurses pass their anger and frustration with physicians onto vulnerable coworkers. This is called "submissive aggressive syndrome." When researchers studied primates, they discovered that when a primate lost a fight, he would walk away and swat another primate who was innocently minding his own business.

Nurses often cite verbal abuse from peers and supervisors as a reason for leaving their jobs. "Researchers report that verbal abuse contributes to 16%–24% of staff turnover and 25%–42% of nurse administrator turnover" (Braun et al., 1991; Cox, 1991; Hilton et al., 1994). In the U.S., "the turnover rate is 33%–37% for clinical practicing nurses and 55%–61% for newly registered nurses. Approximately 60% of newly registered nurses leave their first position within six months because of some form of lateral violence" (Griffin, 2004). In another study, 45% of new-to-practice nurses were humiliated (McKenna, 2003).

In addition, nurses who report the greatest degree of conflict with other nurses also report the highest rates of burnout (Hillhouse and Adler, 1997). In 2001, Dr. Linda Aiken of the University of Pennsylvania's Center for Health Outcomes and Policy Research released a study that examined reports from 43,329 nurses from the United States, Canada, England, Scotland, and Germany. The study found that nurse dissatisfaction was high in all of those countries except for Germany. Burnout and dissatisfaction were reported by 43% of U.S. nurses, and 27.7% planned to leave the profession within a year (Aiken, 2001).

In a nursing shortage, these statistics are especially foreboding and demand that every nurse, on every level, accept the challenge of ending nurse-to-nurse hostility and creating a new culture.

Food for Thought: Exercises

1. Answer this question: Could the potpourri of terms that we have created to describe negative behaviors be an example of the very infighting they describe?

2. Consider this: Nursing theorist Margaret Newman believed that transformation happened through pattern recognition and that shifts occur as the client recognizes their own patterning. If we are the client, what pattern do you recognize within yourself that has the ability to transform your work environment from hostile to healthy?

Summary

The wide variety of terms used to describe negative, disruptive behaviors has hampered our ability to study the problem. Understanding these behaviors along a continuum of harm is not only helpful, but demonstrates how these behaviors can escalate. In this book we will explore horizontal hostility within the context of peer-to-peer relationships between nurses.

The commonly held belief that horizontal hostility is a staff nurse problem is a myth, as these behaviors have been found at all levels of the profession. Stories from the front line are disturbing and along with recent research on prevalence confirm that we do indeed have a problem.

Chapter 2

The Impact of Horizontal Hostility

In the societies of the highly industrialized western world, the workplace is the only remaining battlefield where people can 'kill' each other without running the risk of being taken to court.

—*Namie and Namie,* The Bully at Work

Learning Objectives

1. Discuss the impact of horizontal hostility on 1) the individual and 2) the organization.

2. Examine the relationship between horizontal hostility and patient safety.

According to the Workplace Bullying Institute, the industries most prone to bullying are healthcare, education, and government. Of these three groups, healthcare is the only one in which the smallest error can lead to death, which makes it a high-stress environment. In addition, many nurses miss meals and breaks that typically provide time for them to renew their energy levels and relationships. Time to reflect on the demands of the work environment and opportunities to create a shared story about the important work that we do is rare.

Surveys conducted in 2012 by the Society for Human Resource Management and the Workplace Bullying Institute found that:

- 80% of harassment cases were legal and could only be considered plain cruelty

- 73% of incidents involved verbal abuse

- 62% reported malicious gossiping or spreading rumors or lies about coworkers

- 51% of organizations reported incidents of bullying in the workplace

- 15% witnessed the emotional or psychological abuse of coworkers

Within the past fifteen years, 71% of survey respondents reported experiencing uncivil behaviors (Cortina et al., 2001). Another study focusing on frequency found that at least 20% of survey respondents experienced incivility at least once a week (Porath and Pearson, 2009). Hostile behaviors are a common experience of workers in the United States.

And hostile behaviors are not limited to nurses. These behaviors occur throughout the caregiver spectrum. There is good reason to suspect that bullying behaviors are handed down from the medical education culture. In a study of 2,884 students from the class of 2003 at 16 United States medical schools, 63% reported having been belittled by faculty and 71% were belittled by house staff (Charney, 2011).

Note that horizontal hostility is not limited to females, either. "We saw many instances of [horizontal hostility] in our sample of male RNs. They too made disparaging remarks about colleagues. They too experienced frequent verbal attacks by coworkers. One male nurse spoke of being 'wounded with words.' Another said, 'She purposely attacked me, embarrassing me in front of others, humiliating me, trying to make me look incompetent'"(Thomas, 2003).

As a frontline manager, I have witnessed horizontal hostility on numerous occasions. One nurse would constantly write up other nurses, rather than speaking to those particular nurses directly. It was not unusual for me to come into the office in the morning and find three incident reports in my box targeting the same person. Problems arose because new hires and resident nurses found it difficult to fit into a clique. Comments like "I hate to follow *her*" were common.

The longer the nurses had worked together, the harder it was for others to join their group. Nurses would constantly put down each other by making snide comments, and new nurses struggled to be perfect, knowing that every mistake would be seen as a direct reflection of their competence. Much to my chagrin, the practice of horizontal hostility was quite common on the unit.

Of all the types of aggression that nurses encounter (patient-to-nurse, nurse-to-visitor, doctor-to-nurse, and nurse-to-nurse), nurses report that **the most distressing type of aggression to deal with is nurse-to-nurse aggression** (Farrell, 1999). Such interpersonal conflicts rob us of our energy, deflect our interests from patient care, and prevent us from unifying in order to obtain the resources we need to do our jobs. The consequences of horizontal hostility can be felt on all levels: individual, professional, and organizational.

Impact on the Individual

Bullying behaviors set the course for a lifetime of damage. Duke University researchers interviewed 1,400 children (ages 9–16) about their social lives and then checked in with the same group 10 years later. Children who had been the victims of bullying were four times more likely to have an anxiety disorder; and children who did the bullying were four times more likely to have an antisocial disorder. The most troubled group was made up of the kids who had been both victims and bullies, because they were 14 times more likely to develop a panic disorder and nearly five times more likely to be depressed (Copeland, 2013).

The effects of a hostile work environment cannot be minimized. Research shows that verbal abuse significantly affects the work environment by decreasing morale, increasing job dissatisfaction, and creating hostility (Manderino and Berkey, 1997; Aiken, 2001). Bullied staff reports a decreased sense of relaxation and well-being at work, increased mistrust, low self-esteem, and lack of support from both staff and superiors (Cook et al., 2001). New research validates that nausea, weight gain, irritability, depression, post-traumatic stress disorder (PTSD), and anxiety are experienced by the victims of horizontal hostility and bullying behaviors (Rocker, 2008).

Victims of horizontal hostility experience a wide range of emotional, social, psychological, and physical consequences. For example, the medical community recognizes several physical ailments as being triggered or aggravated by stress: irritable bowel syndrome, migraines, hypertension, allergies and asthma, arthritis, and fibromyalgia. Emotional-psychological damage can be less obvious and can include poor concentration and forgetfulness, loss of sleep or fatigue, indecisiveness, anxiety and nightmares, and obsessive thinking about a bully (Namie and Namie, 2000).

At the October 2005 conference on horizontal violence, Gerald Farrell, RN, PhD, summarized some of the known effects of verbal abuse.

Emotional

- Anger, irritability
- Decreased self-esteem, self-doubt
- Lack of motivation and feelings of failure from being unable to meet personal expectations

Social

- Strained relationships with partner and friends (one-third to one-half of relationships between partners and family members worsen after someone simply witnesses bullying)
- Low interpersonal support/absence of emotional support

Psychological

- Depression
- PTSD—50% continue to suffer from stress five years after the incident
- Burnout—depersonalization, lack of control
- Maladaptive responses—substance abuse, overeating

Physical

- Decreased immune response or resistance to infection
- Cardiac arrhythmias (increased risk of heart attack due to continuously circulating catecholamines)

Recent research supports earlier findings:

- A 2012 study of the psychological consequences of bullying in Australia found that impact varied depending on whether the nurses worked in the hospital or aged care, and full- or part-time. Full-time aged care nurses reported higher psychological distress than part-timers. Hospital nurses reported higher psychological distress, while aged care nurses reported higher depression (Rodwell and Demir, 2012).

♦ A study across four Swedish industries of 4,238 workers from the government's Institute of Environmental Medicine followed witnesses to workplace bullying for 18 months. At the end of the measurement period, women witnesses showed a higher prevalence of clinical depression (33.3%) than men witnesses (16.4%). Simply being exposed to bullying proved to be a significant risk factor in developing depression from negative workplace conditions (Emdad et al., 2012).

♦ More than half of those people who experienced hostility at work reported that they lost time worrying about the uncivil incident and its future consequences. After three studies investigating the objective consequences of both direct and indirect rude experiences, researchers found that both were harmful to task performance. Even a one-time event can affect objective cognitive functioning and creativity (Porath and Erez, 2007).

Seasoned nurses may recall that 20 years ago, new grads were treated as they often are today—harshly, as though they were being hazed to earn membership into the group. But many nurses do not remember horizontal hostility to the extent that it exists now.

Little research documents when this behavior escalated and spread from new grads to staff nurses. Informal conversations seem to point to the late 1990s, when managed care and hospital mergers restructured the healthcare setting. At the time, no one realized the tremendous impact these changes would have on people (Weinberg, 2003). The financial gains promised were never delivered because no one took into account the most critical factor of all: human factors. For example, feelings of identity were threatened, and feelings of fear and loss resulted in serious cultural conflicts. Increased demands on nurses increased their stress levels. During this time period, between two-thirds and three-fourths of all industries, including hospitals, failed to meet their predicted economic gains because the impact of mergers on culture was overlooked (Cartwright and Cooper, 1993; Marks and Mirvis, 1992).

The Affordable Care Act has also impacted nurses as hospitals buy out other hospitals in an effort to stay financially viable. In the current financial model, nurses have been asked to do more with less because hospitals can no longer depend on profit from their traditional revenue streams (e.g., readmissions, overuse, unnecessary surgeries, and highjacking the inpatient chargemaster). As the entire healthcare system is transitioning from volume- to value-based care, nurses have an opportunity to work in interdisciplinary teams, across silos, cliques, and hierarchical levels to directly impact the delivery of care. This will require unprecedented levels of teamwork.

Furthermore, nursing is embedded in a national culture which is struggling with the basic question, "Does everyone have the right to healthcare?" Culture, as we will see in Chapter 4, is critical. It determines what we perceive, and what we don't. And one of the greatest challenges with horizontal hostility is that it is masked in larger cultural issues and cloaked in invisibility.

Organizational Impact

It is imperative that healthcare organizations re-examine workplace concerns with the goal of creating environments that support nurses in their endeavors to provide quality care.

—*Sofield and Salmond (2003)*

Nothing is as destructive to an organization as a toxic work environment. Horizontal hostility creates such an environment by producing feelings of inferiority, anger, powerlessness, and frustration, which are counterproductive when working in a group. Emotional issues will incapacitate even the greatest of initiatives.

Horizontal hostility "is a self-serving, nonproductive response that perpetuates an escalating cycle of resentment and retaliation" (O'Hare and O'Hare, 2004), and research shows that the interpersonal conflict it causes has a direct negative impact on group conflict and work satisfaction (Cox, 2003). Indeed, interpersonal conflicts affect teamwork, patient safety, and quality of care (Leppa, 1996), as well as intent to leave.

The emotional and physical health of employees is a product of the work environment and a key factor in group dynamics. When horizontal hostility enters the picture, it detrimentally affects the environment by producing a host of physical ailments that result in a loss of time from work (absenteeism, time off with worker's compensation, family medical leave of absences) and reduced productivity while at work. These responses affect not only the organization's bottom line, but also the efficiency of the entire facility. Quality is impacted because **there is a perceived inverse relationship between horizontal violence and quality of care: as horizontal violence increased, the quality and safety of patient care decreased** (Purpora, 2010).

The invisible thread that weaves us together is the quality of our relationships. High-quality relationships are reflected in cohesiveness or solidarity—employees who are "all on the same page" and who function with a clear vision of the organization's goals. Researchers have also noted a direct link between high rates of group cohesion and work satisfaction and a lower turnover rate in acute care settings (Amos et al., 2005). Clearly, the hallway conversations that result from such cohesion often give us the critical information and support we need as we do our jobs. Now more than ever, streamlining processes and procedures in hospitals is critical to patient safety and financial efficiency.

The Financial Impact

The effects of nursing stress have potentially enormous financial and human costs.

—Hillhouse and Adler (1997)

"Nursing leaders are becoming more aware of the costs and consequences of hostility among nurses to the healthcare system and to individual nurses" (Arle, 2004). Some economic effects, such as high turnover rates, are obvious. Significant literature also validates the effects of stress and burnout on nurses (Aiken et al., 2002). For example, when positions need to be filled due to sick calls, compensation claims, and family medical leaves of absence, overtime and agency costs accrue. An Australian study published in 1999 in the *Journal of Advanced Nursing* showed that 34% of nurses who experienced bullying took off more than 50 sick days in a year (Farrell, 1999). In addition, the high cost of replacing nurses during a nursing shortage demands that we become aware of the reasons nurses are leaving.

Other economic costs are more difficult to quantify—e.g., the cost of decreased productivity as well as increased mistakes. In the same Australian study, 25% of nurses reported decreased productivity, and 27% reported impaired ability to perform their tasks. Studies confirm that verbal abuse causes a decrease in morale and an increase in errors and staff turnover. But this is just the impact on the victim.

Witnesses to rude behavior report cutting back their work efforts, letting the quality of their work slide, and feeling less committed toward their organization.

A large, diverse national sample found that:

- 47% intentionally decreased time at work

- 38% intentionally decreased work quality

- 80% lost time worrying about the incident

- 63% lost time avoiding the offender

- 66% said their performance had declined (Pearson and Porath, 2009)

Performance losses in other industries have validated the true cost of disruptive behavior. Executives of the Fortune 100 firms reported spending as much as 13.5% of their total work time (seven weeks/year) mending relationships and replacing workers who just can't or won't take it anymore. Pearson and Porath have demonstrated that managers can actually calculate the dollar amount lost from horizontal hostility by providing a cost worksheet and reviewing a corporate case study. They explicitly show that even rare occurrences can create profound associated expenses, as my experiences validate.

In one organization, two bullies on the night shift got away with hostile behaviors for over a decade. Interventions by human resources were constantly thwarted and sabotaged. These senior nurses intimidated new staff, gossiped constantly, and formed a clique that even the FBI could not penetrate. Then one day the director received a petition spearheaded by union members and signed by one hundred nurses demanding immediate removal of all managers from the unit.

The cost? Thousands of dollars in consulting fees, precious time and resources redirected from patient care to monitoring, nurturing, and re-engaging staff over many months, high turnover, painfully decreased management and staff morale, and a massive distraction from patient care. Negative behaviors are more virulent and invisible than C. difficile!

Professional Impact

Retention during a nursing shortage

As the nursing shortage becomes more acute, the reputation of hospitals and of specific units within those hospitals will become more important. Students in their clinical practicums will assess the quality of relationships and decide where they want to work based on their student experiences. Both new grads and floating inter-department nurses will choose to work on nursing units where they feel valued and supported, so creating a healthy work environment will give facilities a proven competitive advantage.

Yet research shows that new grads are at a higher risk for experiencing hostility. New grads are more vulnerable to bullying behaviors and lateral violence because they often lack the confidence and social connections that can ward off negativity (Weaver, 2013). The most recent research found turnover rates of 17.7% the first year, 33.4% the second year, and 46.3% within the third year, with new nurses most negatively affected by interpersonal relationships (Cho et al., 2012).

Exposure to hostility and bullying is one reason that experienced nurses are leaving the profession. Disruptive behaviors directly impact dissatisfaction, turnover, and intent to leave (Simons, 2008). Coworker incivility appeared to be the most damaging and was associated with higher levels of mental health symptomology (Laschinger et al., 2013). In a nursing shortage, the impact of horizontal hostility cannot be ignored. Currently 10,000 people turn 65 every day in the United States. According to the U.S. Bureau of Labor Statistics (2012), the number of employed nurses required to serve this population will increase 26% by 2020—an increase of 712,000 nurses. In addition, 495,000 replacements are needed to replace the current retiring workforce, bringing the total nursing demand to 1.2 million nurses by 2020.

But even as we head toward the worst nursing shortage in history, 40 percent of nursing schools are turning away students due to lack of faculty, and the mean nurse faculty age is 53 years old. Universities cannot compete with the high salaries that an advanced-prepared nurse can earn in the private sector, so the pool of nurses with master's and doctorate degrees will continue to decrease, resulting in a shortage of educators (American Association of Colleges of Nursing).

Ultimately, the shortage comes down to what each of us can control on our own level. As managers, directors, chief nursing officers (CNOs), and educators, we must make it a priority to learn why nurses are leaving our profession.

Patient safety

In a knowledge-based economy, nurses who leave can never truly be replaced, because they have taken with them a vast and unrecorded wealth of information. More than half of employees who are treated uncivilly consider leaving—and one in eight actually does leave (Pearson and Porath, 2009). But while employees may leave, the patient cannot.

There is a direct link between disruptive behaviors and cognition (Porath, 2007) and therefore patient safety. The vast majority of tasks performed by physicians, nurses, and pharmacists are cognitive and require a significant amount of concentration: drawing up, administering, or ordering medicine; assessing medical status, patient progress or plan of care; selecting the right surgical instrument; deciding if the patient is responding appropriately; taking vital signs; etc. Cognition—the ability to think clearly—is critical to the safe delivery of patient care.

In 1999 the Institute of Medicine estimated that 98,000 Americans die a year from preventable medical errors. An updated review based on data from 2008–2011 found that serious harm seems to be 10–20 times more common than lethal harm, and that preventable harm is approximately 400,000 errors per year (James, 2013). Clearly we have not met our primary obligation to first do no harm.

"Disruptive behaviors have a significant impact on team dynamics communication efficiency, information flow, and task accountability" (Rosenstein and Naylor, 2011). In an emergency room study of 370 physicians and nurses, 32.8% of the respondents felt that disruptive behavior could be linked to the occurrence of adverse events, 35.4% to medical errors, 24.7% to compromise in patient safety, 35.8% to poor quality, and 12.3% to mortality.

The effect on teamwork cannot be minimized. Teams that work together well produce a synergy born of respect and trust. Studies of 16 major medical centers revealed that junior surgical teams in small cities and rural areas learned new, complicated procedures faster than teams in medical centers with vast resources, top-notch research facilities, and highly esteemed surgeons. The critical differentiating element that facilitated team learning proved to be **psychological safety**. Negative, disruptive behaviors are distracting, detrimental, waste time and energy, and contaminate teamwork (Porath and Pearson, 2009).

"Simply witnessing rude behavior in the workplace significantly affects our ability to perform cognitive tasks." Just watching other people being treated rudely causes us to perseverate about the event (Porath and Pearson, 2009). Human beings replay the scene in their minds again and again, trying to make sense of why someone would act so differently from other members of the group. This distraction increases the vulnerability of our patients and our chances for making an error. Instead of focusing on the patient, our attention is on the outlier who is demonstrating disruptive behavior.

Disruptive behaviors are more likely to occur in high-stress areas like the emergency department, intensive care, or operating room—all areas where the patient is the most vulnerable. Why is there a direct relationship between high stress and disruptive behaviors? Because the human brain is actually still a reptilian brain, and any threat triggers our flight-or-fight response. In other words, any perceived threat, real or imagined, reroutes our neural pathway to the amygdala where billions of sensory motor stimuli send messages to our brain, and we instinctively react to avoid pain or loss (Donadio, 2012).

To assess the impact of disruptive behaviors on collaboration and communication, the VHA surveyed 4,530 nurses, physicians, and administrators in 2008 and found that 65% of respondents reported witnessing disruptive behavior in nurses. Sixty-seven percent of the respondents saw a direct link between these behaviors and adverse events: the result for medical errors was 71%, and patient mortality, 27% (VHA, 2008).

National calls to action

Our patients will never be safe, unless the caregivers are safe. Until we all feel supported, connected, and valued, we will not have kept our ethical promise to our patients to first do no harm.

The impact of disruptive behavior in healthcare

In a study of 370 emergency room physicians, nurses, and staff, 32.8% felt that disruptive behavior could be linked to the occurrence of adverse events; 35.4% to medical errors, 24.7% to compromises in patient safety, 35.8% to poor quality, and 12.3% to patient mortality. Eighteen percent were aware of a specific adverse event that occurred as a direct result of disruptive behavior (Rosenstein and Naylor, 2011).

In recognition of the detrimental effects of disruptive behaviors, the following organizations have taken a firm stance:

- **2001**: The American Nurses Association Code of Ethics is the professional code for guiding nursing practice. Provision 1 clearly states: "The nurse, in all professional relationships, practices with compassion and respect for the inherent dignity, worth, and uniqueness of every individual ..."

- **2008**: The Joint Commission issued a sentinel alert calling for organizations to "address the behaviors that undermine a culture of safety." The Commission clearly acknowledges that disruptive behaviors are a safety issue, citing concerns about medical errors, poor patient satisfaction, adverse outcomes, higher costs, and the loss of qualified staff. Each healthcare setting must create behavioral codes of conduct and establish a formal process for managing unacceptable behavior, because disruptive behavior is a threat to patient safety.

- **2008:** The Center for American Nurses published a position statement acknowledging the effects of disruptive behavior on patient safety, quality of care, and recruitment and retention of new nurses.

- **2010:** The Center for American Nurses released an updated position statement on disruptive behaviors:
  - "Lateral violence and bullying has been extensively reported and documented among healthcare professionals, with serious negative outcomes for registered nurses, their patients, and healthcare employers. These disruptive behaviors are toxic to the nursing profession and have a negative impact on retention of quality staff. Horizontal violence and bullying should never be considered normally related to socialization in nursing nor accepted in professional relationships. It is the position of the

Center for American Nurses that there is no place in a professional practice environment for lateral violence and bullying among nurses or between healthcare professionals. All healthcare organizations should implement a zero-tolerance policy related to disruptive behavior, including a professional code of conduct and educational and behavioral interventions to assist nurses in addressing disruptive behavior."

Food for Thought: Exercises

1. Reflect carefully on the last two adverse events from your current workplace, and answer this question: Did disruptive behavior of any kind play a role in the process?

Summary

Of all types of aggression a nurse experiences, peer-to-peer hostility is the most hurtful (Farrell, 1999). Studying this issue had been hampered by the lack of a universally accepted definition, as well as by a lack of awareness by staff nurses and leaders that the problem exists. Tales from the front line are consistent with the research and demonstrate the tremendous personal, professional, and organizational impact of this behavior.

Nurses who experience the highest degree of conflict also report the highest degree of burnout (Hillhouse and Adler, 1997). The effects of a hostile environment are reflected in poor patient and employee satisfaction scores and, ultimately, in the reputation of the hospital or academic setting.

New nurses will be drawn to healthy environments; it is therefore imperative that we acknowledge horizontal hostility is a serious problem and learn strategies to intervene.

Resources

Social Intelligence by Daniel Goleman

Odd Girl Out by Rachel Simmons

The Cost of Bad Behavior by Pearson and Porath

Creating and Sustaining Civility by Cynthia Clark

C h a p t e r   3

Exploring Theory

Marie's Story

A manager's point of view

Quitting was heart-wrenching. As I turned the key to lock my office door for the very last time, a thought occurred to me: I was doomed from the first time I ever opened this door. I never had a chance—and I never saw it coming.

It had taken me almost six months to quit because something I just couldn't quite put my finger on was holding me back. I remembered the advice of a wise friend who had said, "You can't close one door and open another until all the lessons have been learned." For months, I had struggled to understand what else I could possibly learn from this job. After seven years working 60 + hours every week managing a large surgical unit, I was frustrated and exhausted. I felt like 90% of my energy was spent just trying to get the resources I needed to do the job "they" expected. Articulating my unit's needs felt like screaming into an echoing abyss. I hadn't exercised in two years and was suffering from every classic symptom of burnout. So why, then, was it so difficult to quit? What was wrong with me?

Then one day, when I was getting onto the elevator, I simply got it. I looked at another manager who was already in the elevator and, as we said our perfunctory hellos, a sickening feeling punched me in the gut. As always, her eyes were riveted to the floor in order to avoid any chance of conversation. Suddenly I remembered a book that I had read a long time ago, Clan of the Cave Bear. In the story, the caveman society decides that Ayla does not exist. No matter how frantically Ayla waves her hands in front of their faces or clutches for her mother's hand, the tribe ignores her. It was society's worst form of punishment because members would die from being ignored.

I looked at the manager's dispassionate face and saw what I feared: I was dying of loneliness. Despite having good relationships with my staff, physicians, and administration, I had been banned by my peers, but I hadn't the faintest idea why. The years of being ignored were taking their toll.

At this point, all I really knew was how I felt. Suddenly, I remembered a story my teacher had told me about Romanian orphans in the 1950s. Hundreds of infants were routinely diapered and their bottles propped up in their cribs, but so many babies were dying that the government sent for a team from the United States to help determine the cause of death. The infants, they discovered, were dying because of lack of touch. And so, before the elevator doors even opened again, I saw myself reaching out through the bars, dying from rejection, from invisibility, due to lack of human touch. The depth of the rejection was the lesson that had been too painful to acknowledge.

I went back to my office with the realization that I could never move into another position at this institution because I was not supported by my peers. I had received absolutely no training, and even if I had, it wouldn't have mattered—I didn't learn the rules until too late in the game. And so I quit. I felt so torn. I really loved my staff.

Oppression Theory

Oppression elicits negative behaviors: silence, a lack of voice, poor self-esteem, and the sublimation of the experience of powerlessness through the internal divisiveness known as horizontal violence.

—DeMarco et al. (2005)

The term "horizontal violence" was coined by theorist Paulo Freire in 1972 to explain the conflict that existed in colonized African populations. Freire observed that an imbalance of power always resulted in the formation of a dominant and a subordinate group. Whenever there are two groups and one has more power than the other, he argued, oppression occurs when the values of the subordinate culture are repressed. This is called the oppression theory.

Freire noted that members of the subordinate group would feel inferior because they were forced to reject their own values and characteristics in order to maintain the status quo. As they acted out their feelings of self-hatred on one another, internal conflict began to spread. The values, beliefs, and characteristics that the colonized Africans had once respected and cherished in themselves were lost.

In 1983, Sandra Roberts, PhD, RN, FAAN, applied oppression theory to nursing and argued that "an understanding of the dynamics underlying leadership of an oppressed group is important if strategy to develop more effective leaders in nursing is to be successful" (Roberts, 1983). She noted that nursing displayed many of the characteristics of an oppressed group: low self-esteem, self-hatred, and feelings of powerlessness.

Founded in a patriarchal society and composed predominately of women, the nursing profession was set up from the start to assume a subordinate position. It is not hard to imagine the circumstances under which the nursing profession originated: In a time when women had practically no rights, nursing provided women with an opportunity to escape their fate and stand on their own. Yet in order for this new profession to be acceptable—especially given that the women would be caring for men who were strangers—nursing was portrayed as a "calling" or as "God's work" (Reverby, 1987). Nurses were viewed as angels of mercy—and angels don't get angry.

From this new paradigm came a set of expectations, albeit unrealistic, that nurses struggled to meet:

◆   A nurse is consistently caring.

◆   A nurse rejects her own needs and works long hours for little reward.

◆   A nurse never complains.

◆   A nurse is always subordinate and speaks only when spoken to.

Significant literature postulates that nursing is an oppressed discipline (Roberts, 1983; David, 2000; Torres, 1981; Daiski, 2004) and that the origins of this oppression can be traced back to gender issues (Kanter, 1979; Farrell, 1997; Reverby, 1987; Gordon, 2005). Hence, nursing is "an oppression by gender and an oppression by medical dominance" (Dargon, 1999), with physicians often assuming dominance over their "subordinates."

The culture of oppression in nursing

"Powerless groups also tend to admire and imitate those they perceive as powerful" (Daiski, 2004). Nurses replicate the traditional power differentials that they perceive in the dominant group. For example, after telling a patient story, a CNO learned that in order to be respected by her peers, she would need to focus on "what is really important"—meaning the financials. This was communicated to her by nonverbal gestures such as frowns and a sarcastic comment.

Nursing leaders in the hospital setting did not consciously select the behaviors of the dominant group. They did what all humans do in a power differential: they imitated the behaviors that would allow them to gain access to resources and power for their nurses. Some of these behaviors are stoicism, intimidation, refusing resources, focus on financials, closed doors, lack of visibility, and giving orders and directives without input. If nursing leaders did not align themselves with the unquestionable values of the dominant group, then they were viewed as "not being a team player."

My director paged me, and when I called her back she was angry and said, "Come down to my office immediately." I was nervous as I knocked on her door. She was pacing back and forth in front of her desk. "Is there a problem?" I said, still wondering what was going on. "Yes. A big problem! Sit down. You are over budget this month," she said, irritated. "And just what are you going to do about it?"

I passed the VP of nursing in the hall about 7 in the morning and she turned to me abruptly and said, "Will you stop by my office on your way home?" By noon, I had to go to the pharmacy for antacids because I couldn't stop worrying and my stomach was churning.

I am a nursing student and school starts at 0700 every Monday morning, but the manager kept refusing my request not to work the Sunday night shift. First she ignored me, then she said I needed to write down the request, then finally, she just refused.

The above scenarios demonstrated overpowering, intimidating behaviors by a CEO, director, VP of nursing, and nursing manager—all unconsciously learned behaviors. But what is even less rarely perceived is the effect on the delivery of safe, quality patient care. Only recently have researchers begun to gather data linking disturbing emotions to patient safety. For example, in a VA study from 2008, Dr. Rosenstein and his colleagues found that over 32.8% of nurses and physicians could link an adverse event to disruptive behavior; 35.8% could link these behaviors to poor quality; and 12.3% to mortality. Our emotional and mental states are intrinsically linked, and a student nurse who is angry and upset cannot deliver optimal care; nor can an intimidated manager be present in rounding to his or her patients.

Any profession that holds a belief system rooted in subordination will feel oppressed, and horizontal hostility is the natural expression of this suppressed anger. Add to the equation the increased pressures incurred by nurses after the restructuring of healthcare in the 1990s (which resulted in a hierarchical organizational structure with little nursing representation), and then again in 2012 (as the Affordable Care Act addresses overuse and access issues), and it is easy to see how horizontal hostility has continued to gain momentum.

Debby is complaining again. As I walk onto the floor, the air hangs with her negativity. "What's the problem, Debby?" I say to her and to the group of nurses all huddled around the main station.

It takes me several minutes to drag it out of her. The problem, it seems, is that a new nurse is not working weekends, and Debby is resentful. "Debby, we have had self-scheduling for more than two years now. If you don't want to work weekends, just change the schedule." She looks at me in shock.

"What do you mean?" she asks, her voice filled with disbelief. "Do you mean that for two years now I could have had every single weekend off?"

"Yes."

Debby does not make a dash for the schedule but instead stands there, flabbergasted, trying to comprehend how or why she did not understand that the prison door was never locked; she could have walked out anytime. Now it is my turn to take in what happens to people when they work in the nursing culture for a long time. The term "learned helplessness" takes on special meaning. Oppression is no longer a buzz word from my theory class.

One of the defining features of oppression is that both the dominant and the subordinate groups internalize the norms set by the dominant group and both groups accept them as normal. After a period of time, no one—not even the subordinate group—notices or questions these unspoken rules (Roberts, 1983).

This pattern occurs today in the behaviors of physicians and nurses. Nurses are not aware of how the dominating actions of physicians—such as avoiding direct eye contact, not bothering to learn a nurse's name, and having only abrupt conversations—keep nurses in the subordinate position (Bartholomew, 2004). What, then, are the behaviors of *nurses* that we do not see, that we accept as normal, and that perpetuate horizontal hostility?

One behavior is that new nurses accept the culture they walk into as normal. As one new nurse said to me, "I was never a nurse before. I thought it was normal for the new nurse to answer call lights for 18 patients while the experienced nurse sat and knitted." As humans we walk into an unknown environment and scan and acclimate to the status quo based on hundreds of years of socialization. Social learning theory supports the strong influence that observation has on learning behaviors:

Learning would be exceedingly laborious, not to mention hazardous, if people had to rely solely on the effects of their own actions to inform them what to do. Fortunately, most human behavior is learned observationally through modeling; from observing others, one forms an idea of how new behaviors are performed, and on later occasions this coded information serves as a guide for action.

—*Albert Bandura,* Social Learning Theory *(1977)*

Horizontal hostility is often accepted as normal and is—in my experience—not consciously committed by the perpetrators, who are aware of their actions, but not of the profound negative effect that their actions have on the victim. One theoretical explanation for this is suppression, which "occurs when thoughts and emotions are either consciously or unconsciously eliminated from awareness. In this way, the individual is protected from overwhelming anxiety or helplessness" (Farrell, 2001).

The nurse may not be conscious of the harm she is causing if she is responding to oppression of which she is not aware.

Powerlessness

When anger is suppressed and cannot be directed upward, nurses lash out against each other.

> There had always been a lot of tension between another manager and myself, so I thought it might be helpful to explain the oppression model to her. When I said that we were an oppressed group and that the backstabbing and low self-esteem we suffered were related to our powerlessness, Margaret vehemently disagreed.
>
> "Do you feel like you have power?" I asked. "Why, yes," she responded. I tried to recall some specific examples. "Remember when the budget was due and if any manager needed more hours of care, we had to take them from another manager because there was only a fixed number of FTEs? It was like a scene from Oliver Twist! There we were, all starving for hours of care, and whoever wanted more had to beg from someone else who was already understaffed!"
>
> Margaret still wasn't convinced. I thought of another example. "We are supposed to round with staff frequently, asking whether they have what they need to do their jobs, but no one would ever dream of ever asking us! Do you have what you need to do YOUR job?"
>
> End of conversation. Margaret stood up and walked away—either she couldn't see the truth or didn't want to.

Our perception of our own powerlessness is the root cause of horizontal hostility, yet the powerlessness itself is so ingrained that we do not acknowledge its role in the social construct of nursing. This invisibility may be closely tied to gender definitions. Power is rejected (on a subconscious level) by the subordinate group because it is viewed as a dominant group characteristic. "Traditional conceptualization of power and caring are presented as polar opposites ... power is congruent with the characteristics of masculinity, whereas the characteristics of femininity prepare women to care" (Falk-Rafael, 1996).

In the oppression model, the values of the subordinate group—in this case, caring—are denigrated by the dominant group and, at the same time, the values of the dominant group—in this case, power and money—are elevated. Unconsciously, the subordinate group pushes away its own values and assumes the values of the dominate group (lean, efficient, fast, etc.). The subordinate group, therefore, is left powerless and with a weakened sense of self.

Such an extreme power differential between the subordinate group and the dominant group creates an undertow with a strength we do not see, and it takes the nursing profession far off course. Margaret has no idea where she is.

Testing theory with reality

No one wants to see themselves as a member of an oppressed group. In order to demonstrate oppression and overcome denial, I use an imagination exercise. The exercise guarantees psychological safety because participants are assured that they will never share the information with others. The only place this confidential exercise happens is in their mind. Over 5,000 nurses have been asked:

> *If I could guarantee you in writing that the conversation would turn out exactly the way you had hoped and planned, is there someone you would speak to at work to create a healthier work environment?*

The answer was overwhelmingly "yes" from all but 15 nurses. The exercise continues:

> *Pretend I ripped up the written guarantee. Imagine the person you need to speak to is sitting next to you right now and you are going to speak to them regardless. How would you rate this conversation on a pain/discomfort scale from 0 to 10?*

Approximately 80% of nurses answered 8–10. This phenomenon is called "self-silencing" (Jack, 1993). Participants are then asked to volunteer the reasons why they have not had the conversation in the past and to share what thoughts or feelings have stopped them from speaking to their colleagues. In over 100 hospitals and conventions across the country at which I have spoken over a five-year period, the most common answers have remained remarkably consistent:

◆ Fear of making the situation worse

◆ Fear of hurting the relationships or someone's feelings

◆ Fear of retaliation: gossip, backstabbing, isolation, warping the message, the silent treatment, a bad assignment, someone refusing to help me

◆ No time

◆ Why bother? Nothing will change anyway

Most audiences will have 2–3 poster sheets of paper covered with responses that stem from fear. These answers represent their lived experiences. A pivotal moment occurs when I point to the audience's list of reasons for self-silencing and ask, *"Who is doing this to you?"*

And a lone voice will always answer softly, *"We are. We do these things to each other."*

This is oppression unveiled: The unconscious acting out of horizontal hostility to each other without the realization that we ourselves are the perpetrators is congruent with oppression theory. By guaranteeing psychological safety, this exercise helps nurses to see through the veil. In addition, the consistent answer "Why bother? Nothing will change anyway" validates the feelings of powerlessness by the oppressed group.

The purpose of the "veil of oppression," as Roberts refers to it, is to prevent us from seeing the truth (1983). This veil is thin enough to see through (we admit among ourselves that some nurses eat their young), yet we do not acknowledge its presence or remove the veil because we don't even realize it's there.

We are creatures of habit and quickly get used to it, like a floater in the eye. The major reason that horizontal hostility is such a threat to our profession is that it is so insidious. We can't fight or even acknowledge a threat to our profession that we can't see. The veil of oppression keeps us hidden.

Why is being invisible so important to nurses?

Invisibility

Five years of being ignored went by, and then one day I finally heard the gossip about me. "Who does she think she is, having a three-day retreat for her charge nurses? Where did she get the money?"

Then one day a peer stopped me in the hall after I had obtained a much-needed 0.5 support position and caught me totally off-guard. "You better be quiet now, missy. Now that you got what you wanted, you had better just keep that mouth of yours shut."

Herein lies the catch-22: At a very primal level, there is an unspoken belief that nursing's identity must stay invisible in order to survive. Like fish that travel in a school to stay safe, all oppressed groups have an understanding at a deep, fundamental level that is never expressed: homogeneity is the key to survival; *in order to survive we must stay together at all costs.* Therefore, when a nurse stepped out of his or her school of fish, to speak his or her truth, he or she was effectively silenced back into the group by the overt and covert behaviors that are now recognized as horizontal hostility.

It is this very invisibility that keeps the group in the subordinate, oppressed position and prevents solidarity. "Infighting within the profession prevents mobilization of resources to confront the larger issues of healthcare reform" (Smith et al., 1996).

The current hierarchical system keeps nurses invisible and subordinate. In her book, *Nursing Against the Odds,* Suzanne Gordon expertly identifies how this invisibility is kept alive—from physicians taking credit for nurses' work to daily failures to acknowledge nurses' contributions. Such a structure causes problems: "Years of invisibility take their toll. When nurses get no positive public credit for their work, [their] sense of professional self-worth slowly erodes" (Gordon, 2005).

In addition, when nurses cannot practice from within their value set, their self-esteem falters. For example, caring—a cherished value—has assumed a position of little importance in today's traditional hierarchical institution; it is difficult to quantify and even harder to fit into the budget. As a result, nurses feel insignificant and undervalued.

From the staff nurse's perspective, the dominant group in healthcare's hierarchical pattern today is primarily administration and insurance companies (from administration's perspective, it is the broken, dysfunctional "system"). Distrust spreads like a virus through an organization because people say that quality and safety are important but then dictate staffing ratios that are unsafe for a particular shift or unit. Money is the top focus for any organization because finances determine if the doors stay open.

> *In Iowa in the early 2000s, Jim eagerly began his tenure in a small community of 30,000 as the new CEO. He immediately saw the need for patient education and began workshops on quitting smoking, losing weight, and managing blood pressure and diabetes. After three years, the board of directors called an emergency meeting. "Jim," they said solemnly. "We have a problem. Our hospital census usually runs around 40, but now we are running at 22. Either stop your community education programs, or you are fired."*

With no control or input into the budget or open access to resources, nurses function as an oppressed group in healthcare's hierarchy. The primary goal of nurses is to provide the highest level possible of quality, safe, patient care. Nurses intrinsically know that their capacity to demonstrate caring, empathy, and support is critical to the patient's recovery and plan of care.

> *I was simply washing an old man's back when suddenly he burst out sobbing. "Did I hurt you?" I said, handing him a box of tissues and stopping the washing. But he responded gruffly, "No, go on now." Finally, after several moments he softly shared, "It's just that my wife died 22 years ago ... and no one has touched my back since." "What was her name?" I asked. And for 20 minutes he told me all about what she planted in the garden, and why she loved the rain. But that's nowhere in my charting.*

> *The experienced PICU nurse had helped couples deal with grief and loss before, but today, the couple seemed especially distraught. He approached the father who shared that they had come to terms with their son's fatal birth defects, but that they were Indians who believed that if their son died in this hospital, his soul would be trapped here for all eternity. So immediately the nurse called the janitor who provided access to an outside court and stayed with the couple until the baby's soul was released to the heavens.*

What is the billing code for an old man's grief or for a free soul?

When the values of the oppressed group are not honored or recognized by the dominant group, then the oppressed group devalues them as well and self-esteem drops. What we offer for free is not valued in a culture where the predominant value is money, and ever so slowly we stop valuing caring ourselves. The values of healthcare, however, are but a shadow of the values of our greater society, as demonstrated in the exercise below. We live in a society that believes that the rational mind, science, and technology trump emotion, art, and caring. The following example is an example of this hierarchy cloaked within our own profession:

> Thirty ICU nurses attending a workshop were presented with a challenge as I pointed to an empty flip chart. "Do you see this white piece of paper? Imagine the white piece of paper represents the nursing profession. If I draw a line on the bottom of the paper, what does that line represent?"
>
> After several minutes a voice from the back said, "Rehab." And so I drew another line just above to which the group answered, "Medical," then "Surgical ... L & D ... Tele ... PICU ... CCU ... ER ... OR ..."
>
> But the group went silent as I drew the last line at the top of the page. "What's at the top?" I queried. No one would answer.
>
> "You are," I said writing "ICU" on the very top line to a group of solemn faces.
>
> Where did this nursing hierarchy come from? If you are the best ICU nurse in the whole world and I am recovering from a multi-injury head-on collision and my brain is mush and I can't remember who I am, I need the best rehab nurse in the world who will stay with me for the 6 to 7 months it takes for me to take my first step—I don't need someone who can run 6 to 7 pumps. But when I am on the precipice of life and death in an ICU bed, then I need the best ICU nurse in the world. There is not one single area of nursing that is more important than another.

The nursing hierarchy as expressed by nurses consistently in the above exercise reflects societal prejudices in that the ICU nurse who uses the most technology is more esteemed than the rehab nurse whose most vital tools are encouragement, insight, and the ability to connect with the patient on a personal level and establish trust.

The organizational hierarchy also invalidates another nursing value: the concept of reflection. In a study published in 2004 in the *Journal of Clinical Nursing*, researchers found that nurses who participated in reflective practice were made to feel that they were outside the norm (Mantzoukas and Jasper, 2004). Yet reflective practice is a key mechanism in understanding and processing our nursing experiences as our patients.

The oppression model thus offers a reasonable framework for explaining horizontal hostility, including hierarchical abuse, clique formation, low self-esteem, and the inadequate response of nurse managers. Under this model, hierarchical abuse is an effort of the dominant group to keep the subordinate group in their place. Clique formation is a survival mechanism—people band together to weather the stress of oppression. Low self-esteem, a known characteristic of any oppressed group, stems from a rejection of core values. And the inadequate response from nurse managers (in dealing with horizontal hostility) most frequently occurs because they have taken on the characteristics of the dominant group.

Weakened sense of identity

I spend all of this time filling out 10 pages of a progress record and not once have I ever seen a physician even look at my charting. After working on the unit for 15 years, I think there's only one doctor who even knows my name.

Our invisibility is a significant contributor to our weak sense of identity. "Evidence that nursing is little known and misunderstood is all around us" (Buresh and Gordon, 2003). In the controversial case of Terri Schiavo, the nurses who took care of Terri were noticeably absent from media discussion, even though they had cared for her for years in her vegetative state. Nurses are not among expert sources quoted in news stories or analyses of mistakes in healthcare (Buresh and Gordon, 2003). Although nursing is the largest profession in healthcare, it is also the quietest—from an organizational standpoint, down to each individual nurse.

Organizational restructuring has removed nurses from key decision-making positions. The average tenure of a chief nursing officer in 2012 was 17 months for a large system of over 400 hospitals—a decrease from 24 months only a year earlier.

Freedom from oppression

According to oppression theory, the oppressed group does not need to overthrow the dominant group to be released from the cultural power dynamics. No rebellion or dramatic uprising is necessary. All that is required to free a group from oppression is:

1. *To lift the veil*—Nurses must realize that the overt and covert behaviors that are defined as horizontal hostility are hurtful individually and collectively, and that these are self-inflicted wounds. We can redirect our power by taking control of our own voices starting with everyday interactions.

2. *To raise our individual and collective self-esteem*—Voice is a synonym for self-esteem. Every time we self-silence, we give away our true power. Self-silencing is group behavior and a reaction to a perceived threat. The self-esteem of nurses will rise as a group as one by one we look into the mirror and acknowledge the profound impact we have on our patients every day—and voice our concerns and opinions to each other and the entire healthcare team.

As was true for the colonized Africans in Freire's study, the cultural identity of nurses has suffered over the years primarily due to the circumstances surrounding its origin. Nursing was born in a patriarchal society and by circumstance placed in the subordinate position. This, combined with the fact that technology and science assumed a greater level of importance in American society, perpetuated the cultural meme that "nursing was soft stuff" and "nurses do what physicians tell them to," or the ultimate meme of all: invisibility, e.g., nursing services are just charged with the room. (Merriam-Webster defines a cultural meme as "an idea, behavior, or style that spreads from person to person within a culture.")

But change is all around us. Many hospitals and systems are now led by a chief nurse who is also the chief executive officer. Organizations like The Truth About Nursing monitor the image of nursing in the media and call our attention to both positive and negative representations of our profession, seeking to raise awareness and advocacy for the clinical training and expertise that nurses provide as autonomous practitioners on the healthcare team.

Several editorials have been written by nurses around the country, most notably by Theresa Brown in *The New York Times*. In addition, the role of nurse practitioner has opened the door for millions to receive direct care primarily from a nurse where patients can witness the skill and knowledge that the nursing profession has to offer firsthand. These are all examples of nurses increasing their presence and voice. Power does not come from emulating the dominant group, but from holding up everything that represents nursing.

In 1981, Jean Watson stated, "While nursing is on its Odysseus-like quest to develop the science of nursing practice, the universal humanistic art of nursing lies unattended." Over 30 years ago, she perceived that the profession was seeking to validate itself by aligning with the dominant group, and she encouraged us to pay equal attention to and validate both the art and science of nursing practice.

The skills to encourage a stroke patient to swallow or the skill set required to accurately monitor central line venous pressure do not compete with each other. One skill is not better than the other. They are complementary skills and equal in value to the patient who is in the bed. We do not have to diminish the importance of caring and connecting with another human in order to elevate the profession. Nursing is both an art and a science, and of all professions, is uniquely positioned to be able to draw from either in the healing of our patients.

> *When we deny, moralize, and sort the good from the bad, some of the dynamic vitality of the image is lost. Repressed content always makes itself known in other ways.*
>
> —*Elizabeth Robinson,* The Soul of the Nurse

Without a unified voice, nurses cannot assume their true role in healing society. Deciding on entry-level college requirements would accelerate this transformation because the general public would then perceive nurses as decision-makers who can function with a single voice. Currently, there are over 500 nursing organizations. None of these organizations alone can impact society in the way that 3.1 million nurses could together.

May I speak with you a minute in private?

The energy between the dominant and oppressed group is always the result of the actions and reactions of both groups. For example, let's look at the unequal power game that occurs sometimes between some physicians and nurses (of course noting that the majority of nurses have good MD-RN relationships). The physician is angry when a nurse calls at midnight to alert him that the patient's pain medication is insufficient (dominant). So the next time she calls, she begins her phone conversation with an apology, "I'm sorry to bother you...," thus lowering herself and playing the game (oppressed). But what if the oppressed nurse didn't play the game? Instead, the next time the nurse sees this physician she says, "May I speak to you for a minute in private?" and gives the physician feedback on the personal impact of the annoying tone of their prior phone call, and on how that tone of voice could be detrimental to receiving critical patient information in the future from other nurses (freedom from oppression).

What is necessary to overcome oppression is awareness, self-esteem, and assertive communication skills.

Supporting Theory: Insights From the Animal Kingdom

Psychological stress and displaced aggression

If a rat is subjected to a stressor such as a series of very mild shocks, he develops a prolonged stress response—his glucocorticoid levels increase, as does his probability of developing an ulcer. However, if the rat is given a block of wood to run over and chew on when the stress occurs, he is far less likely to get an ulcer because he has an outlet for his frustration. If a rat receives a mild shock and there is another rat in the cage, he will "run over, sit next to the rat, [and] bite the hell out of it" (Sapolsky, 1998). **Scientists refer to this as "stress-induced displacement aggression." Nurses refer to it as "eating their young."**

Two other important factors identified in the rat stress studies were predictability and the perception of control over a situation. Whereas unpredictability increased the stress response, *just the perception of control* over a stressor decreased its effect.

In nursing, we lose out on all three counts; we do not have an outlet for our frustration, unpredictability is high, and the perception that we have control is low.

Psychological stress and social support

Primates also exhibit a great deal of displaced aggression. If a male baboon loses a fight, he will turn around and attack a baboon who was just sitting there minding his own business. But scientists have also noticed something else about primates' stress response: Given the exact same stressor, "the primates react differently *depending on who is in the room*" (Sapolsky, 1998). If the others present are strangers, then the stress is worse. If the primate's friends are in the room, then the stress response decreases. Social support networks, therefore, significantly affect how primates handle psychological stress. "Profound and persistent differences in degrees of social support can influence human physiology as well" (Sapolsky, 1998).

The implications for nursing are clear. In the drive for increased efficiency and productivity, opportunities for social support have decreased significantly. For example, when charts were kept at the main nurses' station, communication between both nurses and physicians occurred more frequently and not only about the patient; in general, these were conversations where we built relationships. Decreased social interactions were not an intended, anticipated outcome of moving charts from the nursing station to the bedside.

> *The surgeons round, and I don't even know they've been here. I'd love to discuss the plan of care and ask questions but they round quickly and leave—sometimes before the patient is even awake.*

"Social capital" is a phrase coined by Harvard professor Robert Putnam, who studies the time that we have to connect with each other. In his book, *Bowling Alone,* Putnam points out that social capital is worth more than financial capital to an organization or industry. For example, when a manager with a great deal of social capital asks a nurse to work an extra shift, the answer will likely be "yes." The manager has garnered social capital from supporting this nurse on other occasions, and so the nurse reciprocates.

> *I was scheduled to work Christmas and I have three small children under 12. I never even asked. The week prior to Christmas the manager offered to work day shift for me since she has teenagers.*

The impact of low social support at work is compounded by the fact that social capital has decreased tremendously in our broader society (Putnam, 2000). The very fabric of our interactions is changing rapidly. Multigenerational, professional, and informal community group participation has decreased as time spent online has increased. Participation in community activities has decreased as Facebook time online has increased. Research shows that there is a significant difference between an online connection and a bond. People who spend more time on Facebook have been found to have significantly lower family support (Marche, 2012). People are forming virtual communities where they may never actually see each other—especially with gaming. Today there are more than 183 million Americans gaming, five million of whom play over 45 hours every week.

Technology's impact on social isolation and lonelines

For those who use computers outside of work, we have increased our average use of computers for leisure from 12 minutes to over 1.5 hours a day (Wallsten, 2013). But there hasn't been a flat one-on-one tradeoff because watching television, cuddling up on the sofa to watch "Walt Disney's Wonderful World of Color," or listening to "Pagliacci" were all communal activities, compared to our solitary computer/iPad/Google Glass world. The statistics are dramatic:

♦ Each minute we spend online is correlated with 27% less work time, 28% less time on other leisure activities, 5% fewer physical interactions, and 12% fewer minutes sleeping

♦ People living alone in 2011 comprised 28% of all households as compared to 17% in 1970

♦ In 1950, 10% of households had one person; in 2010, that number rose to 27%

♦ In 1985, 10% of people had no one with whom to discuss important matters

♦ By 2004, that number rose to 25%

Loneliness has increased dramatically over the last five decades. A 2010 AARP study found that 35% of adults older than 45 were chronically lonely, as opposed to 20% of a similar group only a decade earlier—an estimated 60 million people. As nurses we know that loneliness affects our patient's physiology, and this has now been confirmed by research. The morning urine of lonely people has higher levels of the stress hormone epinephrine (Cacioppo, 2008). For people older than 60, loneliness is a predictor of functional decline and death (Perissinotto, 2012). When these societal influences against social capital are combined with the financial influences pressing for higher efficiency in hospitals, the double whammy is profound and measurable. Our social support networks both at work and at home are clearly lacking, contributing to an increase in psychological stress.

Humans as social animals

Bees construct hives out of wax and wood fibers, which they then fight, kill, and die to defend. Humans construct moral communities out of shared norms, institutions, and gods that they fight, kill, and die to defend.

—Jonathan Haidt

For generations, humans have held themselves as separate and above the animal kingdom. If we looked at ourselves as the social animals that we are, and understood our automatic responses, motivations, and physiology, we would advance as a species in leaps and bounds.

In his book, *Predictably Irrational,* Dan Ariely cites numerous examples of just how irrational humans can be. When offered two dollars if they will sign a form giving their soul to the devil, the majority of atheists refuse to sign. When we are offered candy with a check, we give a higher tip. If we are standing outside of a Cinnabon store, we are three times more likely to give change for a dollar. And in all of these situations, we are totally unaware that we are behaving as social animals.

"Reason and emotion are not separate and opposed. Reason is nestled upon emotion and dependent upon it" (Brooks, 2011). We are not the rational beings we imagine. Fear immediately channels resources from high brain regions to the amygdala. *Cognition, rational thought, and logic are suspended even with mild anxiety and stress.* Our behaviors, conscious or not, are triggered by our emotions.

Neuroscientists have found that emotions that govern behavior are biologically based. Anger, fear, shame, indignation, jealousy, pride, compassion, gratitude, sorrow, and joy appear to be part of an overall program of bio-regulation (Clippinger, 2007). The conscious mind gives itself credit for things it really didn't do and concocts tales to create the illusion it controls things it really doesn't determine at all.

The human brain

The mid-brain, or mammalian brain, is strongly involved with emotional reactions related to survival. It functions as our emotional gatekeeper and contains the amygdala: a highly sensitive arousal system that responds to sensory and motor stimuli. A multitude of hormones and complex neurotransmitters communicate constantly to keep us safe by avoiding pain and danger, acting without our conscious forebrain's thinking process. The mid-brain has been doing this for 200–300 million years (Donadio, 2012).

- We do not think, "I am going to roll my eyes at her when she comes over here."

    We *feel* annoyed because someone is on our turf or in our space.

- We do not think, "I am going to sigh now to show her who is boss."

    We *feel* personally or professionally threatened.

- We do not think, "I'm going to fold my arms in this staff meeting to show my manager I don't care what she/he says and I will not listen to a word they say."

    We *feel* defeated, defiant, or angry.

And that is the problem. *We do not think.* We feel as our five senses take in the circumstances and we react in nanoseconds. The vast majority (if not all) of our overt and covert behaviors are triggered by our primitive biological programming that was designed to keep us safe. Even the smallest stressors rewire our neurological system back to the amygdala. That's why rational, cognitive approaches to behavioral change can provide structure and tools to work with … (but) when it comes to making sustainable changes, emotions trump cognitive thoughts hands down" (Donadio, 2012).

Applying this information to the phenomena of horizontal hostility is illuminating and eliminates the stigma and shame attaching hostility to our profession. When overpowered, human beings unconsciously direct their energy toward each other in the delicate dance of power that plays out in everyday workplace dramas, following a design that was set in motion when we were primates. We trust and cooperate more readily with people who look and sound just like us—and take only 170 milliseconds to decide if another person is in or out of our group.

These are all behaviors of the social animal called humans.

Populations at Risk

Bullies scan groups for the weakest. Maybe it is an evolutionary remnant of our place in the animal kingdom. All predatory species select and attack the weakest prey.

—Namie and Namie, The Bully at Work

Whether a new hire, a transfer from another department, or a new resident nurse, any member introduced into a powerless group is at high risk for experiencing horizontal hostility. Horizontal hostility is a learned behavior that historically has been used by groups with low self-esteem to break in new nurses—or in terms of oppression theory, to acculturate them into the group. These are learned behaviors used to teach our unspoken rules. If the status quo is rocked in any way, fear escalates and expresses itself as horizontal hostility. It's as if "until she is one of us, she is a threat." The last thing new nurses need today, however, is a difficult rite of passage.

While new graduates are easy prey to horizontal hostility, nurse managers are also extremely vulnerable targets, due to their marginalization and relative isolation from each other. In other words, nurse managers do not typically feel at ease eating lunch with the staff nurses they supervise or the administration to whom they answer. Therefore, this group has a particularly weak identity unless championed by a strong nursing administration and given the time and resources necessary to build solid team-oriented relationships.

Marginalized groups tend to take on the characteristics of the dominant group. This pattern might explain the comments staff nurses make about new nurse managers, such as, "She is always in her office doing paperwork," "She's one of *them* now," or "She has no clue what is going on in the floor because we never see her."

Managers or staff members are especially vulnerable if they act differently than other members of the group because their behavior inadvertently draws attention and threatens the group's invisibility. Like the child of an alcoholic parent, a nurse sees his or her invisibility as a means of staying out of harm's way and out of the spotlight. Unnecessary attention puts the entire group in danger—it doesn't matter if this attention is for the good of the group. Thus, a manager who excels, complains, dresses differently, etc., is immediately perceived as a threat *at the most primal level* because she is standing up to the dominant group. His or her actions run the risk of retaliation by the dominant group against the entire subordinate group.

To prevent this from happening, the subordinate group immediately demonstrates behaviors that will cause that nurse to leave the group (see Figure 3.1). Gossiping, backstabbing, ignoring, etc., are all means toward this end. These behaviors, designed to extricate the nurse from the group, are biologically wired and considered vital to the survival of the group.

> *You wouldn't think it would happen to a director, but they ran her out. They sabotaged her and ignored her until she quit. That one only lasted a year. I could see how they distanced themselves from her. She always sat alone.*

> *The managers were supposed to have lunch together on Thursdays. It was supposed to be a time where we could confide and find strength and camaraderie. I only lasted two weeks and never went back again. Somehow every word I said made it back to my director.*

Why Is Horizontal Hostility So Virulent?

Denial

The strongest force that perpetuates horizontal hostility is denial—denial by both the nurses who are committing the hostile behaviors *and* the targets who are keeping silent. When any behavior has been a part of a culture for a very long time, it is perceived as normal. So normal, in fact, that hostile behaviors are not labeled as bullying behaviors. In this way, the organiztion hinders its own responsibility to act (Martin and Klein, 2013).

Witnesses also play a role in perpetuating horizontal hostility. For example, senior nurses witness overt behaviors intended to diminish new nurses on the unit; what they see matches their own orientation, so they don't identify the behaviors as a problem. All the players in this drama—the organization, the victim, the perpetrator, and the witness—fail to acknowledge the problem or take any action.

| Figure 3.1 | The 10 most frequent forms of lateral violence in nursing practice* |

1. Nonverbal innuendo (raising of eyebrows, face-making)
2. Verbal affront (covert or overt, snide remarks, lack of openness, abrupt responses)
3. Undermining activities (turning away, not available)
4. Withholding information (practice or patient)
5. Sabotage (deliberately setting up a negative situation)
6. Infighting (bickering with peers)
7. Scapegoating (attributing all that goes wrong to one individual)
8. Backstabbing (complaining to others about an individual and not speaking directly to that individual)
9. Failure to respect privacy
10. Broken confidences

Ordered from most to least frequently encountered.

Adapted from Duffy, 1995; Farrell, 1997; McCall, 1996; McKenna, Smith, Poole, & Coverdale, 2003. SLACK Incorporated and The Journal of Continuing Education in Nursing. Reprinted with permission.

Hostility's invisibility

In addition to hostility being accepted as the norm, hospital restructuring has significantly increased the manager's scope of practice, making these distruptive individuals less visible than ever before.

> *I had four units! There was supposed to be a supervisor in each of those units, but a year went by and no one had applied for the position in three of the units. So there I was trying to get the schedules out for 300 people. It was insane. I worked 12–14 hours a day and weekends.*

This increased workload has significantly decreased the manager's presence on the unit, as managers struggle with the paperwork (incident reports, budgets, schedules, position requisitions, etc.) for multiple units. The system was not set up to support the manager. Thus, hostility has become even less visible to the only person with the power and authority to interrupt it. The manager is now noticeably absent.

Ineffective supervisor intervention

She was like gangrene. I told the director that she was infecting all of us, but still she [the director] did nothing. I told her again and again. Finally, people started leaving, and there was a mass exodus. She just wouldn't cut her off so that we could all live.

Managers have been accused of not responding appropriately to staff concerns about horizontal hostility. "Nurse managers are blamed more for acts of omission than for acts of commission" (Farrell, 2001). Many nurses who complain to their managers do not feel like it makes any difference (Farrell, 2005).

Managers may fail to respond for several reasons: their assimilation into the dominant group, a heavy workload, poor conflict management skills, inadequate education or role modeling, feelings of helplessness (or lack of support), and an underlying perception that hostility is the norm. In a study conducted by Gerald Farrell, PhD, RN, for his PhD dissertation at the University of Tasmania, Australia, Farrell found that respondents' main concern about nurse managers was "their failure to implement supportive structures when incidents arose or to take appropriate action to prevent their recurrence" (Farrell, 2001).

However, sometimes the greatest obstacle for a manager is the Human Resources department itself. Designed to protect the employees and ensure fairness, the pendulum has often swung too far in the other direction:

Everyone knew this employee was a drain on the team with his absenteeism and tardiness. So I made up a Performance Improvement Plan. After the written warning was in place for 90 days, the employee wasn't absent or late a single time—until day 91.

Without support from the system, managers are set up to fail and are perceived by staff as ineffective when, in fact, they have followed every step of the policy, only to be undermined by HR policy on "day 91." Now, as hospitals tighten their budgets in order to financially survive healthcare reform, once again the span of control for managers is being expanded as history repeats the cost-cutting measures of the late 1990s.

The supervisor as the bully

Abuse from those in supervisory or management positions is referred to as bullying because of the uneven power gradient. The supervisor, in this case, takes on the dominant role and exerts his or her power over staff, and thus oppression is set in motion from a direct supervisory level. Managers have been reported to use primarily covert behaviors such as refusing time off or vacations, assigning a difficult patient after a nurse calls out sick, or ignoring nurses entirely. Overt behaviors include providing poor evaluations, writing up an employee for disciplinary action, and excessive vigilance or monitoring of an employee's work.

It doesn't seem to matter if the abuse is vicarious (not directly experienced, but delivered secondhand, as in a rumor) or directly experienced. Both personally and vicariously experienced supervisor abuse has a negative impact which is heightened when both types are present (Harris et al., 2013).

Note that managers themselves report oppressive tactics from their directors, etc.; the pattern is repeated throughout the hierarchy. "A change in the oppressive social structure of hospitals may be needed to truly address horizontal violence in the best interest of the quality and safety of patient care" (Purpora et al., 2012).

Lack of confrontation skills

I asked the charge nurse to come into my office with the staff nurse at the end of the day because they were both so angry and upset with each other. Suddenly, the charge nurse started to cry and quickly covered her eyes with her hands.

"Would you like to do this at another time?" I asked.

"No," she responded. "I'll be okay. Just give me a minute. It's just my alcoholic father—stuff from childhood," she said, composing herself again. "Go on …"

Nurses frequently demonstrate a passive-aggressive communication style; some speculate that this is due to childhood experiences in which one parent abused a substance. From childhood, they bring the message that "Herculean measures should be attempted rather than ever rocking the boat." Maintaining the status quo becomes equivalent to avoiding conflict at all costs. The innate desire to care for others may have also emerged from these childhood experiences—used to "taking care" of things at home, they were drawn to nursing as a profession.

Historically, the most common way nurses address conflict is avoidance; and the most common communication style is passive aggressive. "The profession was founded on silence," (Roberts, 1983) which then became a cultural meme.

Thus, charge nurses who have been on the unit for many years may lack leadership skills—specifically, confrontation/conflict management skills—because of the passivity they developed in childhood. And without supervisory constraints in place, horizontal hostility goes unchecked. Staff continue their behavior without consequence and a toxic culture takes hold.

Today, many people are going into nursing as a second career because they find the profession meaningful and rewarding. These second-career nurses bring with them a variety of communication styles. In addition, new nurses are often more outspoken and assertive and are role modeling healthier ways of communicating. Memes are not stagnant, but constantly evolving. As each nurse speaks his or her truth, our communication meme of silence mutates like DNA as it responds to environmental stimuli and pressures.

Pressure relief

When we vent, we release pressure. Over the past decade there has been a tremendous increase in the pressures felt by the nurse. The human adaptability theory, which states that incremental increases in pressure over time go unrecognized, allows pressure to build up without notice.

Pressure comes from the fact that length of stay has decreased, patient acuity has increased, the weight of patients has increased, and the average age of nurses has increased. Nurses may reluctantly admit that they "were blowing off steam" when they acted out against a coworker.

A nurse who had worked on our unit several years before returned to apply for an evening position. Before interviewing her, I gathered some information from staff who had worked with her in the past. "Is she a good nurse?" I asked.

The nurses responded that, yes, she was clinically sound, but that she was "extremely negative." They did not want to experience her negativity again.

During the interview process I relayed the acceptable and unacceptable behaviors on our unit, when suddenly she interrupted me.

"Wait," she said emphatically. "It's only natural for a nurse to vent; it's a part of the job. When you are frustrated, you have to let it out."

"No," I responded. "That is not our culture here. If you are frustrated on our floor, you have two options:

1. Talk directly to the person you are frustrated with in private, or
2. Come and talk to me."

I was not surprised when she withdrew her application a week later. Hiring for values and articulating the group's norms in the hiring interview gives managers a head start on leading a healthy workplace culture and offers job applicants an opportunity to see for themselves that your unit will not be a good fit.

Professional denial and shame

What is hidden in the unconscious keeps the nurse from accounting for behavior like aggression and compulsivity, which shows up as sabotage, manipulation, and workaholism. It is easier to project denied aspects onto others than to admit our own.

—Elizabeth Robinson, The Soul of the Nurse

It is hard to admit that nurses could be so mean to each other. The foundation of our work is caring. But, as pointed out earlier, caring is not a value honored by the dominant group. It has been diminished in the power struggle that exists wherever there is a hierarchy, and so we then devalue it ourselves. Working in an environment that does not honor caring lowers our self-esteem and creates a great deal of moral dissatisfaction—and this unhappiness unconsciously triggers hostility.

Professional denial is most evident in feelings of shame—a powerful emotion which hides the problem. The roots of the word "shame" are thought to come from an older word meaning "to cover." Horizontal hostility is the shadow side to the profession—repressed and concealed because it is such a polar opposite to the love and caring we see demonstrated by nurses to their patients. It is the complete opposite of the angel meme, and so we distance ourselves from it. But as Elizabeth Robinson says, "Repressed content always makes itself known."

I was asked to give a speech on the topic of healing nurse-to-nurse hostility. But the nursing director asked if I could call it something else. She suggested "Creating

Healthy Relationships"—and 10 people showed up. "I learned my lesson," she said after the presentation. "If I called it 'Why Nurses Eat Their Young,' there would have been standing room only!"

An example of oppression

While visiting an operating room in a major city, I spoke to three different nurses who all complained about immoral, unethical, and unnecessary surgeries. Their stories were poignant and specific:

We put a pacemaker with an exterior battery pack into an 85-year-old man who was so demented that he kept trying to dial out on the battery pack because he thought it was a cell phone.

We put a triple VAT into an 87-year-old women —I can't believe they would do this!

We did a total heart transplant on a 32-year-old man after every other hospital in the city refused to do it because he had failed the psych evaluation. We kept him for over 300 days, but he died after he went home because of the reasons cited in the psych eval—no support system and no will to live after his mother died. But we made money charging for all of those days and that surgery for sure.

Within two hours, at least one (if not all) of these nurses went and "warned the physicians" who stormed into the CEO's office demanding to practice without being scrutinized. Since these physicians brought in over $30 million a year in revenue, their request was granted and the status quo was protected. Even moral distress was trumped by the nurses' fear.

Intermittent reinforcement: Aggression breeds aggression

One of the critical forces keeping horizontal hostility in motion is intermittent reinforcement (Farrell, 2005). B.F. Skinner, the noted behaviorist, discovered that the strongest way to reinforce a behavior was not continuous reinforcement but rather intermittent reinforcement. Sporadic and surprise verbal attacks thus create a hyper-vigilance—if one does not know when hostility will strike, one will always be on guard.

Not only is hostility sporadic, but it is rarely demonstrated by a large number of nurses. The majority of nurses demonstrate professionalism. Because only a few nurses overall are hostile, we tend to think we work in great environments and that if we keep to ourselves, they will not bother us. However, research shows that even one bad apple will destroy trust in the group (Felps et al., 2006). Hostility spreads with the same virulence of a virus if not addressed quickly and efficiently, because bad feelings are more contagious than happy ones.

Being abused is a vicious cycle that leads to increased levels of hostility. That is, "once aggression arises, it is likely to be maintained unless remedial action is taken" (Farrell, 1999).

Food for Thought: Exercises

1. Cognitive-Motivational Relational Theory (CMR) states that we make meaning out of events that happen in our lives by using a two-step process: A *cognitive* response which evaluates why something happened, followed by an *affective* response. In short, we experience an emotion (Bunk and Magley, 2013).

   - Apply this model to a specific event that disturbed you at work. Describe the event, your thoughts, and your feelings *at the time the event happened*.

   - How long ago did the event happen? Write down your current thoughts and feelings about the event.

2. Appraisal theories of emotion state that emotions result from people's inter- pretations and explanations of their circumstances (Aronson, 2005). Use the exercise below (described earlier in this chapter) to apply theory to practice.

   - If you had a written guarantee that the conversation would turn out exactly as you had hoped and planned, is there someone in your workplace you would have a conversation with to create a healthier, happier, and safer workplace?

   - If you answered "yes," can you identify specifically what thoughts and feelings have prevented you from having this conversation earlier?

3. From your observations and experiences, create your own theory explaining the phenomenon of nurse-to-nurse hostility.

Summary

The nursing group will never elevate itself from the subordinate position as long as it is invisible. And the only way to become visible is to:

- Lift the veil of oppression. Nursing leaders must acknowledge the oppression and powerlessness and illuminate the hostility.

- Elevate the self-esteem of nurses individually and collectively (Roberts, 1983).

The oppression model provides a working conceptual framework for understanding horizontal hostility in nursing. It not only explains why horizontal hostility exists, but, more importantly, holds the key to breaking this vicious cycle of aggression.

On a very practical level, the key is to:

- Hold staff accountable for hostile behaviors

- Insist upon a crucial conversation between both parties when any nurse experiences hostility

Time and time again, my experience has shown me that the behaviors stop as soon as the perpetrators comprehend the damage they are causing. It is the very understanding of these dynamics that will result in nurses reclaiming their power and ultimately healing our profession.

Resources

Changing Behavior by Georgianna Donadio
The Social Animal by David Brooks
A Crowd of One by J.H. Clippinger
The Righteous Mind: Why Good People Are Divided by Politics and Religion by Jonathan Haidt

Chapter 4

A Root Cause Analysis of Horizontal Hostility

1. List two extrinsic and two intrinsic factors that add to nurses' stress.

2. Illustrate the concept of work complexity from a recent personal experience.

3. Define "culture" and give one example from your workplace.

4. Examine the impact of 12-hour shifts on nurses' relationships with each other.

Marie's Search for Answers

A new administrator arrived at the hospital, and when she heard a piece of gossip, she immediately called me to her office. The current rumor was that I knew some "insider information" about a restructuring process and that I wanted my position posted as soon as possible. Neither was true.

"Then why the misinformation?" she asked. My heart fell. "It's the culture," I replied sadly, wondering if she would believe me. I didn't even want to believe me! But I couldn't find any other reason or pretend everything was okay any longer.

The administrator encouraged me to find out how the gossip began. I immediately called the manager who had started the gossip and arranged to go up to her office. Clearly upset, I told her what had just happened. Then, for the first time, I got to hear the gossip that had been circulating about me for seven years. I so appreciated her candor and her willingness to share. But why didn't anyone check things out? Why did no one talk to me—for seven years?

During our conversation, the manager would recall a past situation and relay the gossip, and then I would explain what had really happened. As soon as she saw my pain, she saw the truth. It was a powerful and emotional confrontation that ended with her promising "to stop the talking."

I could not hold back the tears as I walked out of her office. I felt transported back to the sixth-grade lunchroom. The work we were both doing was so very, very hard, and this whole time we could have been supporting each other—as if the challenges of healthcare were not enough! It felt like I had found a cure for a disease that had already killed me. It was too late—I had already given my notice. Even crucial conversations with all of my peers could not erase seven years of backstabbing. I felt defeated. I felt cheated.

Through exit interviews and conversations with the administration, I managed to better understand my situation before my last day (I was lucky, for many nurses leave feeling incomprehensible alienation). Inadvertently, I had discovered the unspoken behavioral expectations inherent in the nursing culture. But it took me a long time to not take the rejection personally—I beat myself up about it for months. I try to tell myself that our group was just trying to survive, but some days it takes more convincing than others.

Marie's look back: A reflection interview

What did you mean by "I never had a chance" and "I never saw it coming?"

Marie: *People who had been there for years had the power to smear you and did so before you even knew it was happening. It's like walking into a very important game where the stakes are really high (i.e., my job and feeding my kids), and the people you are playing with won't let you see the rule book. I hadn't realized nursing was so competitive. Lots of poker faces.*

What did you learn in your exit interviews that was helpful?

Marie: *That there was a piece of truth in this situation for me, too. I realized that I had never felt supported in my life and that I probably was projecting that* *to others. When I got past the pain, I was able to acknowledge the support I did receive from lots of other departments—just not nursing.*

I stopped beating myself up because [other nurses] wouldn't let me in. I learned that it was only partly my responsibility to leverage myself with my peers—nursing administration had a responsibility to stop the gossip, but they let it continue, even when they knew it wasn't true. They didn't seem to recognize it for what it was. Nor were they aware of the damage.

I learned that my expectations were unrealistic and that a lot of my frustration had come from trying to work too hard to get the resources I needed. I should have monitored my energy better. At first, I didn't realize the constraints of working in a healthcare institution. Then I wholeheartedly believed that things would get better—and later, I couldn't accept that they didn't.

What were the rules that you didn't know but wish you had?

Marie: *Don't do anything to set yourself apart.*

Don't rock the boat in any way. Silence is golden.

Don't trust ANYONE, ever. NEVER let your guard down.

Never talk to anyone higher than your boss.

If someone has a problem with you, you will never know it—but everyone else will.

If you can't join a clique, you won't survive.

Individual context

After I read Marie's story to a university professor, she responded, "I feel that way too. I try to connect with my peers, but everyone is so busy. The one meeting I do have each week with a colleague is strictly business—there's really no connecting on any meaningful level."

Together we reflected on the pressures that come not just from the university, institution, and nursing unit, but from all directions. In addition to stress generated by conflict with peers, nurses bring a host of extrinsic factors into the situation: the damage caused by poor physician-nurse relationships, disenfranchising work practices, and an increasing demand for higher productivity.

Looking at ourselves and identifying some of the intrinsic factors that foster our isolation and alienation—inadequate conflict management and communication skills, a belief system that does not match reality, a Type A personality, unmet expectations, and burnout—is a good place to start. Because horizontal hostility is a complex subject, understanding all of these perspectives will give nursing leaders the information they need to find solutions.

Intrinsic Factors

- ◆ Emotional state—anger, burnout
- ◆ Personality style
- ◆ Beliefs and expectations
- ◆ Inadequate communication and conflict management skills
- ◆ Generational differences
- ◆ Diversity and racioethnic differences

Our emotional state

All too often we leave the workplace bone tired and soul weary, trying to shake off the sticky residue of moral distress, that awful realization that we could not give patients the care they deserved.
                              —Sandra Thomas (2004)

Anger

Our anger is an expression of our pain. It "is not channeled into constructive actions. It eats away at us inside and takes its toll. It spills over to our own peers, corroding relationships" (Thomas, 2004).

Jackie had been mad for weeks, but no one quite knew why. She just kept writing up people and pointing out omissions in charting. Some staff jokingly referred to her as "the charting Nazi." It got to the point that nurses evaded her constantly, and then overtime increased as nurses took more time with their charting in order to not be punished by being written up.

Sandra P. Thomas, PhD, RN, FAAN, and professor and director of the PhD program in nursing at the University of Tennessee in Knoxville, has studied women's anger for more than 15 years and has conducted studies with both men and women in nursing for more than a decade. In her research, Thomas found that women's anger involved a confusing mixture of feelings. She discovered that when women turn their anger inward, they feel helpless and powerless. However, when women *externalize* their anger they *still feel powerless* because they view an outburst as a lack of control.

What precipitates this anger?

◆ Unfair or disrespectful treatment

◆ A lack of reciprocity in relationships (Thomas, 2004)

We pay a high price for this anger: fatigue, physical health problems (cancer, obesity, and heart disease), depression, and substance abuse. We must stop the harm we are causing to ourselves and learn how to transform our anger into productive energy that will improve our working relationships—and our own well-being.

A recent study of 843 direct care hospital nurses found that nurses under 30 years of age were more likely to experience feelings of agitation and less likely to employ techniques to manage their feelings. The authors recommend that experienced nurses serve as emotional mentors and that we recognize the emotional demands inherent in our work. Understanding the emotional work of nursing is a key factor in understanding burnout (Erickson and Grove, 2007).

Burnout

"Forty percent of hospital nurses have burnout levels that exceed the norms for healthcare workers, and job dissatisfaction among hospital nurses is four times greater than the average for all U.S. workers" (Aiken et al., 2002).

In his book, *Overcoming Secondary Stress in Medical and Nursing Practice*, Robert Wicks specifically addresses the unhealthy culture of healthcare. He defines secondary stress as the pressure that results from reaching out to others in need (e.g., caring for sick patients), which is a constant and continuous reality in medicine, nursing, and allied health. Wicks breaks secondary stress into three components:

◆ Chronic secondary stress, also known as "burnout"

- Acute secondary stress, also known as vicarious post-traumatic stress disorder (PTSD)

- Other unhealthy aspects of the job unique to the medical healthcare culture

There are multiple manifestations and causes of burnout, but there is one common denominator: "a lack that produces frustration" (Wicks, 2005). For nurses, this lack is felt most acutely in the difference between the care nurses believe they should deliver and the care they actually can deliver. Frustrations abound as nurses struggle to obtain the supplies and resources they need to do their jobs.

Other examples of deficiencies surrounding burnout can be the lack of:

- Breaks

- Sufficient staffing

- Professional and personal recognition

- Education

- Coping mechanisms

- Staff harmony (Wicks, 2005)

In the first phase of burnout, individuals begin to experience emotional exhaustion. Their sense of satisfaction decreases, and they feel drained of energy. These signs and symptoms are "brief in duration and occur only occasionally." In the second phase, nurses develop negative ideas about their patients, coworkers, and themselves. When symptoms become more stable, last longer, and are tougher to get rid of, burnout has progressed to stage II. By the time a caregiver has reached stage III, symptoms are chronic and a physical illness has developed (Wicks, 2005).

As I read through the definition and causes of burnout, I couldn't help but wonder: Is horizontal hostility actually a synonym for stage II burnout? The major signs and symptoms are familiar: disillusionment, pervasive feelings of frustration or apathy, and intermittent periods of a week or more of feeling irritated, depressed, and stressed. These are the symptoms I observe among my own staff.

Personality style

What personality types are drawn to nursing? In a 1990 study of self-attitudes and behavioral characteristics of Type A and B personalities in female RNs, researchers found that 82% of nurses classified themselves as having a Type A personality (Thomas and Jozwiak, 1990). The Type A personality is characterized by hard-driving behavior patterns. Individuals with this personality type are typically very driven (often workaholics), somewhat impatient, and aggressive.

In the study, "Type A nurses scored significantly higher than Type Bs on questions about intense job involvement, speed/impatience, and competitiveness." The researchers also found that "Type A nurses are bringing some attitudes and behaviors with them to the workplace that could kindle angry emotions" and contribute to interpersonal relationship conflict (Thomas and Jozwiak, 1990).

"In summary, the Type A nurses appeared to be engaged in competition with time and themselves, as well as competition with other people" (Thomas and Jozwiak, 1990). One observation made today is that admittance to nursing schools is so competitive that college admission officers are selecting the cream of the crop: Type A students with >4.0 averages. This results in a profession that lacks a healthy variety of personality types.

Personal characteristics

A randomized, national study of 1,400 early-career registered nurses found that nurses reporting all levels of abuse were statistically more likely to be female, white, married, English-speaking, in good health, and without young children. Half of this sample reported being on the receiving end of some degree of abuse. They were also more likely to work in a hospital setting (not an ANCC Magnet Recognition Program® (MRP) hospital), in a direct care role, and working 12-hour shifts. It is no surprise that these nurses were more likely to report a lack of supervisory support, lower levels of group cohesion, fewer promotional opportunities, and fewer nurses than scheduled on most shifts. The lack of access to resources (staffing, mentoring, and professional advancement) is representative of a lack of power (Budin et al., 2013).

Belief and expectations

Belief systems

Changing behavior is predicated by a change in our belief system, but education rarely encounters this very deep and personal area. In examining our beliefs and expectations, we delve deeper into the causes of frustration in the workplace.

The following are some beliefs that nurses hold:

- I must have approval from others.
- I must be perfect and feel inadequate if I make a mistake.
- People should be blamed and punished when they do wrong.
- Unhappiness is caused by external circumstances beyond your control.
- You should worry over possible negative events constantly.
- The influence of past events can never be changed or removed.
- For every problem, there is a perfect solution that must be found (Thomas, 2004).
- Compliments are self-aggrandizing.
- Talking about my specific role in the care plan is narcissistic.
- A good nurse should be able to function on her or his own, without any help.
- There is nothing I can do about the situation—that's just the way it is around here.

What does anger have to do with beliefs? Significant correlations have been found between anger arousal and many irrational beliefs (Thomas, 2004). That is, when beliefs don't match reality, we often get angry. When emotions are displaced, misunderstood, and not acknowledged, this anger, as well as a cascade of other conflicting emotions, can escalate into horizontal hostility. The following scenarios illustrate the problems that can arise when our beliefs contradict one another and the reality that surrounds us.

Perfectionism: "A good nurse never makes a mistake."
Justice: "Nurses should be punished for mistakes."

It is 2:50, and Martha is in my office just 10 minutes before the start of her shift, complaining. Martha tells me that I need to get rid of a new nurse who "does not know what she is doing." She makes no qualms about her intentions—Martha believes that it is her responsibility to oust this new employee in order to uphold the standard of care on the unit.

Ironically, I have a quality variance report on my desk about Martha, who forgot to give Coumadin® to one patient last night and forgot to chart it for another. This fact does not faze her. She sees absolutely no connection between the other nurse and the fact that she herself is human and has made a mistake as well. Her response to the drug error is, "Oh." Martha continues complaining vehemently about the other nurse. Her belief that nurses must be perfect, and her inability to see her own faults, is unwavering.

Suffering: "A good nurse doesn't mind suffering."
Self-reliance: "A good nurse will never need help."

Alice is in my office for her performance review. I am really struggling with this one. She is an excellent clinical nurse—the best on the floor. But her negativity is toxic, and staff are weary of her constant complaints. "She brings everyone down," they lament.

During the review, I praise her clinical abilities and then pause. Alice is stoic. I can see the wall.

"One more thing, Alice. As you know, I have asked your peers for feedback, and they are very worried." I reframe her peers' complaints. Half of the wall crumbles.

"You seem so unhappy," I say. "Is there a problem?" Tears flood away the rest of the wall. Out comes Alice's belief system. That a nurse should be self-sufficient at all times. That asking for help is a sign of weakness. That suffering is next to sainthood. That she should be able to handle everything herself, all the time. "I thought that's what a good nurse was," she says.

Our beliefs are formed from our values. But these are not our values. They are the values the dominant group has forced upon our nursing culture: perfectionism, independence, judgment, low self-esteem, and helplessness. **Daily experiences reinforce our belief systems.** Clearly there is an opportunity for nursing leaders not only to bring irrational belief systems to light but also to instill a new set of beliefs based on a new paradigm of an empowered nurse.

For example, governance councils led by frontline nurses in many hospitals now identify issues and brainstorm solutions. These groups support, promote, and validate nursing's role in the plan of care. This structure, created and endorsed by leadership, is a constructive, positive place to solve problems and elevate clinical practice. Another example is TCAB (Transforming Care at the Bedside), which is a template for change initiated by frontline staff and trialed at the individual and then unit level. This framework was created by the Robert Wood Johnson Foundation and the Institute for Healthcare Improvement (IHI) to initiate improvements in medical-surgical units and has had promising results.

Unmet expectations

Years ago, I read a study in *Psychology Today*. The cover page had caught my eye. "What is the most depressing place to live in America?" I thought for sure that the answer would be a very poor part of the country. I was wrong.

Researchers found that the Philadelphia Tristate region was populated by the most depressed people at that time. The reason was because, as young adults, this population expected to have a different lifestyle than their parents—they expected to exceed their parents' lifestyle. But their expectations were dashed as reality—the high cost of living and a slowing economy—set in. This huge gap between what they expected and what actually happened caused the highest degree of depression.

Coming out of nursing school, our expectations of a nurse's job often present a stark contrast to the reality of nursing. As in the story above, it's not the worst-case scenario that produces the greatest depression—it's the large gap between expectation and reality. Marlene Kramer (1974) found that new graduates experience a reality shock that can manifest as hopelessness and dissatisfaction, and that these feelings are often a prelude to conflict.

Today, nursing leaders are investing in transition programs that coach and mentor new-to-practice nurses for up to a year in order to set expectations and minimize shock. These programs address cultural issues that new nurses encounter and provide an open, supportive dialogue that maintains a healthy sense of self-esteem. Outcome data from over 6,000 residents who participated in a year-long, structured, clinical-immersion residency was evaluated over 10 years and it was found that increased competence and self-confidence decreased intentions to leave and decreased actual turnover (Ulrich et al., 2010).

Inadequate communication and conflict management skills

Fear of confrontation and conflict

Anne opens the door to my office. "The patient in 42 says she has not had a bath in two days."

"Well, who had the patient?" I ask.

"Dana."

"Is Dana working today?"

"Yes," she says flatly.

"Well, why don't you ask her about it?"

Now Anne's forehead is all scrunched up. She is not happy. She had already made up her mind (without realizing it) that Dana must have done a poor job. I can hear the judgment in her voice. "What am I supposed to say?" she asks.

"The same thing you just said to me. You say, 'Dana, can I talk to you for a minute? I just came out of 42 and the patient says she has not had a bath in two days.' "

Anne lets out a small groan and leaves reluctantly, as if going for a root canal.

Last year, we had our first charge nurse retreat. It was wonderful. Never before had we been able to simply enjoy each other's presence. On the unit, every conversation seemed to be about staffing shortages or solving patient problems. The retreat, however, gave us the time we so desperately needed to value and appreciate one another.

On this retreat, one of the most amazing eye openers for me, as well as for the charge nurses, was the "leadership cards." In this exercise, nurses selected 20 cards (from a pile of 60) that listed the leadership skills they felt they needed to improve most. The nurses were then asked to pick from this stack of 20 the top three cards they believed would make the biggest difference in their role as charge nurse. Even though all the nurses worked individually for this exercise, all 11 charge nurses picked the same card: "Dealing with conflict." Later that day, we did an exercise and went around the room asking, "What drains you? What are circumstances that rob you of your power?"

I try to hold staff accountable, but some respond so aggressively—they get so angry that it is difficult for me to even approach them ... so I don't.

When I see the nursing assistants sitting down and the nurses running around totally overwhelmed, it makes me angry—can't they see? I feel like a nagging mother hounding children all the time. And that doesn't feel good.

The last time I told an employee that there were way too many personal phone calls at the desk, she punished me! She made my life miserable for weeks by being cold and indifferent.

Me. I drain me. I put such incredible pressures and unrealistic expectations on myself.

There was a unanimous consensus. Everyone felt that his or her confrontation skills were inadequate. Even the thought of conflict made them cringe, and they had no idea what to say or how to say it. Charge nurses did not have the skills to hold staff accountable. Cohesiveness increased dramatically among the nurses as they identified this common denominator and realized that dealing with conflict was an attainable skill. To further emphasize the critical importance of communication, we referenced the AACN standards for a healthy work environment, which state that we must be as proficient in communication as we are with our clinical skills.

Self-silencing

The imaginary exercise on passive communication in Chapter 1 is used to demonstrate how nurses give their power away by their decision to be silent. Speaking up is simply not worth the risk. But this characteristic is not unique to nurses. By listening to stories of women's depression, Dana Jack found that women silence themselves in order to cultivate and maintain intimate relationships (fear of hurting another's feelings, fear of making the situation worse, or fear of losing the relationship (Bartholomew, 2004). She found that self-silencers value the people they work with more than anything else. This value system may be rooted in gender and based on the primordial power dynamics between men and women. Women who witnessed bullying over 18 months showed a higher prevalence of clinical depression (33.3%) than did male witnesses (16.4%) (Emdad et al., 2012).

But why would nurses value peers over patients?

1. Because the majority are women. And for time immemorial women have hardwired into their biology that they need each other to survive.
2. Because in a fear-based culture, the top priority is safety. And psychological, social, and emotional safety are biologically linked to physical safety.

Like fish traveling in a school to stay safe, they are constantly aware at all times of their distance from each other. When I asked a critical care nurse to express how she felt to her peers she responded, "Are you kidding? It would be a feeding frenzy! To say how I feel is like bleeding among sharks ... I would be dinner!"

This is how we learn to keep silent—because past attempts to connect were rewarded with being ignored, the silent treatment, gossip, or being "dinner." The social animal that we are is shaped by overt and covert culturally learned behaviors. This critical care nurse is not working on a team. Teams are characterized by high trust and open communication. In a team, she would be valued, protected, and most of all, safe.

Extrinsic Factors

There has been a revolution in medicine concerning how we think about the diseases that now afflict us. It involves recognizing the interactions between the body and the mind, the ways in which emotions and personality can have a tremendous impact on the functioning and health of virtually every cell in the body. It's about the role of stress . . .

—*Robert Sapolsky,* Why Zebras Don't Get Ulcers

Extrinsic factors include:

◆ Violent workplace—verbal abuse from patients, families, and physicians

◆ Poor nurse-physician relationships

◆ Task and time imperatives—work complexity

◆ Demands for efficiency/productivity

◆ Culture

A violent workplace

Assault rates for healthcare workers are higher than any other industry, with nurses and patient care assistants' experiencing the highest rates of violence (Gates et al., 2011). The United States Department of Justice recorded 429,100 violent crimes against nurses on duty from 1993–1999. "Nurses experienced workplace crime at a rate 72% higher than medical technicians and at twice the rate of other healthcare workers" (Thomas, 2004).

The emergency room is especially challenging. A study published in the *Journal of Emergency Nursing* in 2002 found that 88% of hospital nurses reported verbal assault and 74% reported being physically assaulted while at work by patients, family members, or visitors in the past year (May and Grubbs, 2002). More than half of emergency nurses reported having experienced physical violence and/or verbal abuse from a patient and/or visitor during a seven-day period, with 62% experiencing more than one incident *(NCVRW Resource Guide, 2014).*

Why are family members and visitors so angry? The most common reasons for assault included enforcement of hospital policies (58.1%), anger related to the patient's condition (57%), long wait times (47.7%), and anger related in general to the healthcare system (46.5%) (May and Grubbs, 2002). Nurses have no control over any of the above issues, but they take the brunt of the anger for them from patients, family, and visitors. Clearly in this type of environment we must at the very minimum depend on the camaraderie and support of our physicians.

Poor nurse-physician relationships

Poor nurse-physician relationships affect morale, patient safety, job satisfaction, and retention (Larson, 1999; Rosenstein, 2002; Baggs et al., 1999). A 1997 survey published in the *Journal of Professional Nursing* showed that 90% of nurses had witnessed six to 12 unpleasant incidents between physicians and nurses within one year (Manderino and Berkey, 1997). After reviewing the results of that survey, VHA West Coast—a division of VHA, Inc., a national network of community-owned hospitals and healthcare systems—surveyed 1,200 nurses, physicians, and executives (Rosenstein, 2002). Their results showed that 92.5% of respondents had witnessed disruptive behavior, which confirmed the findings of previous studies.

Have our relationships improved over the last decade? In 2010, nurses, physicians, and staff in an emergency department setting still found that 57% witnessed disruptive behavior by physicians and 52% witnessed disruptive behavior by nurses, and these behaviors had a significant impact on team dynamics, communication efficiency, information flow, and tasks (Rosenstein, 2010). We know that collegial and collaborative relationships with physicians are more common in MRP hospitals than a comparison group (Kramer, 1974). Despite a growing awareness that our relationships with our physician partners impact patient safety, disruptive relationships still exist and there is a great deal of work to be done. Strong leadership is needed to lead the cultural change from a hierarchy to true teamwork both from managers and senior leadership. A single event can shut down communication with a physician for an entire career, affecting thousands of patients by putting them at a greater risk for error.

It is no surprise that the most common feeling a nurse experiences after an incident of verbal abuse is anger (Araujo and Sofield, 1999). **The term "submissive-aggressive syndrome" is often used to describe the fact that nurses who feel robbed of their power (submissiveness) often react by overpowering others (aggressiveness).** There is no healthy outlet for this anger, so it is seldom expressed except through horizontal hostility. But this form of expression creates a new problem and fails to handle the primary emotion: hurt (Bartholomew, 2004).

Task and time imperatives

I said to the nurse, "Mrs. Rather needs a bedpan." But she had no idea who Mrs. Rather was, even though the shift was almost over. The nurse looked at her notes and then finally said, "Oh, 942."

An overload of tasks and time imperatives results in a depersonalization of care. "A nurse's work shift is not finished until all assigned tasks are completed. The nurse who fails to complete his/her tasks at the end of a shift is persona non grata (an unwelcome person) to oncoming shift-worker colleagues" (Farrell, 2001).

Time and task imperatives are so strong that nurses themselves get trapped in them (Farrell, 2001). The focus becomes "what" has to be done in "what" amount of time, and the "who" loses value as tasks accumulate. "So powerful is the notion of task and time imperatives in the nurses' psyche that patients are sometimes seen as *tasks*, not people" (Farrell, 2001). Because of this, we start seeing each other as obstacles instead of human beings. Thus, the new nurse is "in the way." And a nurse has so much on her mind that she refuses help offered to her when she really needs it because to give away a task is to give away control of an extremely delicate operation—her shift.

Even managers, whose jobs are to streamline efficiency, get caught in the cyclone of activity on the floor and therefore cannot see the complexity of work practices clearly. For example, the morning labs on our unit were drawn around 7 a.m. When the physicians came to the floor, their lab results were not ready, so nurses would call physicians in their offices, or interrupt them in the middle of an operation, just to give them a hematocrit value—on every patient. This practice disrupted the physicians and the nurses, so physicians would often keep nurses on the telephone on hold. Because I was either out on the floor helping the staff or in my office buried in paperwork,

it took me two years to see the obvious and to develop a solution: draw the labs at 5 a.m. And then there was the issue of the keys to the patient-controlled analgesic machines—three keys for seven nurses.

Issues like these are just the tip of the iceberg. We are so caught up in what needs to be done that we never get a chance to step back and reframe the picture.

Work complexity

Work complexity is characterized by multiple goals, unpredictability, and constant change. Patricia Ebright (2003) and her colleagues found eight patterns that contribute to work complexity: disjointed supply sources, missing equipment, repetitive travel, interruptions, waiting for systems of processes, difficulty accessing resources, inconsistent communication in care, and breakdowns in communication.

Up to 40% of a nurse's work is not related to direct care (documenting, learning new technologies). Nurses are interrupted mid-task an average of eight times and experience 8.4 work failures per shift while completing tasks that each take only 3.1 minutes (Tucker and Spear, 2006). The average nurse performs over 160 tasks in an eight-hour shift, with each task taking less than 2:45 seconds; and 7–8 items stacked at any given time to perform (Krichbaum, 2007). Our units and hospitals are not set up to support the nurse, and the result is often frustration.

We have adapted to the additional stressors in healthcare very poorly: We have become experts at workarounds. We have lists of backdoor phone numbers and can pull any drug we need from the highly computerized Pyxis machine because we have memorized where that particular drug is (after several incidents of not being able to get the drug when we need it). While these tactics save time, they also increase the probability of committing an error. In haste, we do not double-check our work.

It should not be a major struggle to obtain admission orders for a new patient, stat medications, or a wheelchair for discharge. But it is. Although not necessarily a direct cause of aggression, strict adherence to task/time imperatives "provides the backdrop for situating the occurrence of poor staff relationships within a nursing context"

(Farrell, 2001). The amount of work we must get done within a particular time frame and our lack of control greatly contribute to our psychological stress.

Increased efficiency = decreased reflective practice

Nursing today is much too often like working in a "M*A*S*H" unit, with the exception that there is never any time to debrief. At the end of their shifts, nurses spend two minutes reporting the clinical signs, symptoms, and plans of care for their patients. They do this for four to eight patients and then walk out the door—with all of their thoughts and emotions still flaring.

This lack of time for reflection and connection does not allow nurses to make sense of their emotions and leads to isolation, as we believe ourselves to be alone in our anger, depression, frustration, etc. We suffer a tremendous loss when we don't make time for reflective practices and don't listen to ourselves and others. Exchanging our stories would strengthen our bonds and unite us, but instead, we go to battle every day for years without the debriefing that would save our mental health. This lack of connection fosters isolation. When we don't see others in the same boat, we think, feel, and become life preservers, just looking after ourselves.

Pat is the charge nurse and, at 7:45 a.m., is already in her manager's office venting. "And Kim is still mad! What else am I supposed to do?"

A few hours later, her manager is rounding and runs into Kim. The manager is direct. "I heard you have a heavy load but that Pat can help you." Kim looks overwhelmed, so the manager asks if there is anything she can do.

"Yes," she replies. "You can listen to me."

As Kim's story unfolds, the manager learns that Kim's nursing assistant did not show up until 8:15 a.m. and that no one had mentioned to her that she was going to be late. Kim explains that she then asked a preceptee to hang the blood, but the preceptor said her preceptee already had enough experience, etc.

"I'm sorry," the manager replies. "Let's meet with Pat after the shift."

But Pat does not want to meet. She is very tired and near tears, and all she wants to do is go home. Eleven surgeries have rolled back on the floor, and she is worried about her son, who is away at college. She is frustrated because she cannot make things better. It just seems like it never ends, and the support she offers to others is worthless. Kim, however, insists, and the two come into the manager's office.

Kim is the first to start. She tells Pat how much she respects her and that she thinks the world of her and her leadership skills, but that she is really mad that no one told her that Jennifer, her nursing assistant, would be so late. As it turns out, Kim is angry with Pat because of this, but instead of telling her, she complained about another assignment.

Pat had no idea about Kim's true complaint. She heard the secretary say, "Jennifer will be late," but thought she meant Jennifer the educator, not Jennifer, Kim's nursing assistant. In turn, Pat became angry because she had worked so hard to make a fair report and provide resources yet was treated so harshly.

The conversation only touches the surface. Strong feelings of betrayal lie underneath.

The next layer reveals that Kim was angry about attending a preceptor workshop that Pat had signed her up for that same day. Out comes another story—the real reason behind all the conflict of the day. Angrily, Kim explains to Pat, "It was passive-aggressive of you to sign me up for that preceptor class because you thought I was awful."

As the manager asks what she means, more gossip rises to the surface. Kim had heard a rumor that she was too hard on the new preceptees. So if that was true, why were we sending her to a preceptor workshop—was it some kind of joke? So much pain...

In this debriefing, both nurses had the opportunity to express themselves, and the end result was a great deal of understanding and empathy for one another. It was clear that Kim felt devalued and unrecognized for her precepting on the floor. And she was hurt. The rumblings of the day signaled a much larger emotional issue. Everyone on the floor was aware of the drama and its impact on the atmosphere of the unit, but emotions were so strong and everyone was so busy that the issue was avoided. Had this conversation never happened, an undercurrent of anger would have permeated the floor for weeks or even months. The destructive effect on morale and teamwork would have been horrendous.

The impact of 12-hour shifts

Florence Nightingale said, "Time is the most valuable of all things." On a very practical level nurses need time to work out conflicts in interpersonal relationships, and to do this we need time to be with each other. The increased compression of the workload combined with 12-hour shifts has shortchanged nurses of the opportunity to converse and reflect on the tremendous value of their work to each. Nurses have lost a tremendous amount of social capital.

> *At the end of my shift I met a peer when we clocked out. That was the first time*
> *I saw her because we have bedside reporting and my pod was in the back corner.*
> *I was shocked that I could work an entire shift with my friend and not even know*
> *she was there. But we were so busy …*

Twelve-hour shifts were created as a recruiting tool to a generation of nurses who sought a better work-life balance during a nursing shortage. The problem is that nurses stopped socializing after a 12-hour shift because they were tired—and they didn't want to come into work just to chat on their days off either. Our socializing patterns changed. Without an opportunity to share conversations that were more personal in nature (e.g. "My marriage is on the rocks," "My son was just diagnosed with autism"), our understanding of each other's lives decreased. Without knowing why a fellow nurse is acting negatively, is frustrated, or is performing sloppy work, we tend to judge rather than elicit compassion.

In addition, nurses accrue a considerable sleep debt while working successive 12-hour shifts with accompanying fatigue and sleepiness. Extensive caffeine use was noted to compensate for the average 5.5 hours of sleep 12-hour nurses received (Geiger-Brown et al., 2012). The effect of cumulative fatigue cannot be minimized, as fatigue and burnout decrease our attention span (vigilance) and increase the chance for error. Researchers also found a direct correlation between longer shifts, higher levels of burnout, and patient dissatisfaction (Witkoski-Stimpfel et al., 2012). The challenge for leaders is that 80% of nurses from four states were satisfied with these scheduling practices (Witkoski-Stimpfel et al., 2012). If we refuse to see or admit the damage that 12-hour shifts have done to our patients and ourselves, then we are putting the entire profession at risk.

Culture

Alas, culture is not what we say, what we think, what we mean,
or even what we intend; it's what we do.

—Jon Burroughs, MD, healthcare consultant and educator

Anthropologists say that talking about your own culture is like a fish talking about water; it's the last thing we see because we are surrounded and immersed in it every day. Culture is not written down, everyone knows it, and no one ever says it out loud. For example, the hierarchy in nursing is not written down, everyone knows it, and it remains unspoken, yet it drives many "I'm better than you" behaviors.

As I rounded on the PICU I discovered that there were three pods. On the first pod were all the new-to-practice nurses; on the second pod were nurses with 5–10 years' experience; and at the last pod (closest to the bathroom and the break room) were all the experienced nurses. Did no one notice? Not the manager, the physicians, or the nurses themselves? If one of their own children was admitted, did they not realize that they would insist on a bed on pod 3?

There is nothing more powerful than culture. Not even knowledge or education can compete. In a study of 26 labor and delivery nurses, 78% said they would increase the dosage of Pitocin to the wrong amount if the physician asked them to do it (Lyndon et al., 2011). The hierarchical culture of healthcare has had a profound impact on utilization of best practice and is the antithesis of teamwork.

I decided not to order the overhead bed frame because the patient was going home in just six hours after a microdisectomy (one day postop). Assembling the frame is time consuming, takes additional personnel, and it didn't make sense to go through all that time and effort for a patient to use it only once then go home. When the physician arrived on the floor, he yelled loudly, "Do you understand what an order is? You disobeyed my order!"

Our profession was designed to mimic the military model. Even our terminology reflects it: surgeon general, charge nurse, discharge, and postop orders. In phenom-enological interviews, military metaphors permeate the conversations. Nurses described themselves as "under assault" in a hostile environment (Smith et al., 1996). I can recall a nurse on our floor looking at her schedule and upon realizing that she would be on duty for all three days of our JCAHO visit said, "I want combat pay"—only half joking.

Autonomy

The key drivers of motivation for all humans are autonomy, mastery, and purpose (Pink, 2010). In the military model, nurses lack autonomy to make independent decisions. Autonomy (control over practice) has been shown to be the most important factor in job satisfaction for nurses as well (Dunn, 2003). Physicians give inconsistent responses to nurses who demonstrate autonomy. Depending on the severity of the situation or the time of day, nurses are either applauded or condemned for their independent problem-solving actions; the same physician who applauds a nurse for not calling at midnight will turn around and chastise her for exercising independent thinking during the day. This inconsistency discourages nurses from acting autonomously and leads to hyper-vigilance (Gordon, 2005).

It is very important to note how the pattern of ambiguous or conflicting responses from physicians filters down through the nursing culture. For example, nurses have reported feeling coerced into working "voluntary" overtime by their managers. Another peer-level example is when an ICU team decided not to wake up stable patients for vital signs when sleep was perceived as critical. This decision was left to the discretion of the nurse. Yet in the morning report, fellow nurses would glance upward or sigh if the night shift didn't have the 4 a.m. vitals, thus sending a disapproving, nonverbal vibe that the nurse was just lazy. This, the overpowering message flows insidiously down the chain of command.

Each profession's unique culture is impacted by other cultures. The military model is not attractive to nurses because it squashes autonomy, which is key to job and staff satisfaction. However, awareness of the use of the authority gradient can mitigate its influence.

The entire profession will ultimately benefit from the culture of nurse practitioners because of their autonomy in making decisions and collaborative physician working relationships, which elevate our cultural image. According to the Bureau of Labor Statistics (2012), there are over 105,000 independent nurse practitioners in the United States, and this number is predicted to consistently rise due to the impending shortage of primary physicians.

Culture change

Steve Klasko, MD, MBA, at the University of Southern Florida, believed the only way to change the DNA of the physician hierarchy was from the very start: in medical school. So if you walk into the simulation lab at USF, you will be unable to distinguish career paths because medical students, nursing students, and physical therapists all identify themselves as "a health sciences major."

The "no feedback" culture

In addition, the nursing culture has historically lacked a constructive way to give feedback. Nurses who have worked with each other for 20 years have never been asked to give feedback about their peers, charge nurses, or managers. Because we are human beings, if there is no way to give constructive feedback, we often turn to offhand comments as the only way to express our opinion. Professionals, however, solicit the input of their peers in order to obtain as much information as possible, so that they can more accurately perceive themselves and identify areas for improvement. The very act of asking for this information debunks the myth that we are perfect.

In a high-trust environment, peer review is a valuable tool for growth. The expectation is not perfection. Staff look forward to learning more about themselves, and understand that their peers have important information that they need in order to succeed. Leadership also asks for feedback because it is part of the culture of continuous learning and improvement.

Leadership asking for feedback: One example

Four orthopedic surgeons approached their nurses with a form asking for feedback. Next to their names were three columns entitled Approachability, Patient Complaints, and Professionalism. They asked the nurses to please rate them on a scale from 1–5 so that they could improve—a phenomenal example of leadership that affected the entire surgery center by debunking the hierarchical meme that physicians are humans who somehow do not make mistakes.

Asking for feedback is challenging in a low-trust environment. Staff have reported that the peer review process was sometimes misused as a systematic sabotage system. If a nurse wasn't liked, then nurses would gather in the break room, gossip, and coordinate harmful comments. You can build trust by using peer reviews in two ways.

1. *Ask for feedback on yourself.* Use the same questions below and write down the answers so staff know that you are taking the information seriously, setting an expectation, and leading by example. By doing so, you send a strong message that no one is perfect. Simply the act of asking for feedback has a dramatic impact on the culture and diffuses the traditional hierarchy.

2. *Ask for immediate data.* For example, while gathering feedback for a charge nurse retreat, I offered to watch each nurse's patients while she/he took three minutes to fill out a form. The quick, honest assessments were extremely helpful to the charge nurses. The vast majority had never heard a compliment from a peer about their work before and valued the information. The last questions on the form were open ended:

    – What do you like the best about this charge nurse? (or manager or nurse …)

    – What would you like to see more of from this charge nurse?

Your unique culture

While general observations can be made about the nursing culture, they apply in varying degrees because each hospital has its own unique culture. Yet even within each hospital, departments and even different shifts in the same department have their own unique set of norms. (Float nurses in any hospital will readily validate this fact.) Your culture is a compilation of everyone who has ever worked on that unit, most notably, past leadership.

When behaviors are tolerated over a long period of time by both management and peers, they become acceptable. The only way to change cultural norms is to speak up (*voice = power*). As pointed out earlier, nurses who have tried to do this alone are often experience even more hostility, as they are perceived as a threat to the group's safety on a primal level. Strong leadership from senior administration, directors, and managers is needed to create and maintain a culture of teamwork and mutual respect.

One hospital system listed "Respect" as one of its top four values. The chief medical officer called asking for advice on how to handle rude behavior by two surgeons. But the next day he called back again saying, "I can't do this. I'm not sure the *system has my back. These surgeons bring in a combined $30 million a year." And so I offered him another choice.*

"You don't have to address the rude behavior," I said, as he sighed. "There is another option: Just remove 'Respect' from your core values."

Without the organization's mission, vision, and values aligned with staff's actual behaviors, an organization lacks institutional integrity. **Integrity is born of trust which can never exist as long as there is one exception to the rules.** It is vital to remember that the goal is not to eliminate the person but rather to eliminate the behavior and illuminate the impact that the behavior is having on the entire healthcare team.

Food for Thought: Exercises

Social Epidemiology? A public health researcher at Michigan State University's School of Criminal Justice decided to examine murder through the lens of public health. The study looked at murder as an infectious disease and found that the incidence of homicide spreads much in the same pattern: spiking in a region and then spreading to nearby cities. "To spread, an infectious disease needs three things: a source of infection, a mode of transmission, and a susceptible population." The researcher also found some areas that were resistant to homicide, despite being surrounded by a high murder rate, and will direct future research to examining why these areas appear immune. (Zeoli, 2013).

Answer the following questions:

1. What implications might this research have for explaining horizontal hostility?

2. If we continued to explore along the same lines, what is the source of infection, mode of transmission, and susceptible population for your workplace?

3. If hostility does spread like an infectious disease, what can you do to create immunity in your current work environment?

Summary

Intrinsic and extrinsic factors play major roles in perpetuating horizontal hostility. Horizontal hostility may have its roots in oppression, but there are clearly other forces that fan the flames: a violent workplace, disenfranchising work practices, emotional angst, verbal abuse from physicians, Type A personality traits, unrealistic beliefs, unmet expectations, a culture of no-feedback, and poor confrontation skills.

Although horizontal hostility occurs in all service-oriented industries, it is especially virulent in healthcare. After examining the intrinsic and extrinsic factors that add momentum to normalized behaviors, our focus now turns to a broader context: horizontal hostility in the context of the organizational structure, our profession, and our world.

Resources

AACN standards for a healthy work environment: *www.aacn.org/WD/HWE/Docs/ HWEStandards.pdf.*

C h a p t e r   5

Enlarging the Landscape

Many of our assumptions about human nature turn out to be wrong precisely because they don't account for context … we're more influenced by the actions of those around us than we'd like to believe.

—*Sam Sommers,* Situations Matter

Learning Objectives

1. Explain one way in which the current system is designed to support the invisibility of nurses.

2. Illustrate the conflicting values of the dominant and oppressed group from your work experience.

3. Discuss how the organizational structure enables oppression.

To view horizontal hostility solely in the context of an individual nurse on a nursing unit is limiting and one-dimensional. In order to recognize all the factors that contribute to hostility, we need to expand our focus and examine hostility in three separate yet interwoven contexts: the organizational context, the professional context, and the context of our world. Only by looking back and enlarging the landscape to create and embrace a holistic vision can leaders develop the wisdom and compassion they need to create a culture of respect.

Context Is Critical

Barely six months into my tenure as nurse manager, a sentinel event occurred which directly linked horizontal hostility to medical errors. This single event enlarged my personal landscape and proved to me beyond a doubt that my patients would never be safe unless the nurses themselves were safe and that my role as a nurse leader had to expand to accept the responsibility for creating and monitoring the atmosphere in which my nurses worked just as much as creating and monitoring their clinical competence.

On morning rounds I was informed that a patient had been found with an oxygen saturation of 52% and taken to the ICU at 7 a.m. An MRI showed anoxic changes of the brain that were so significant that the physician was concerned his patient would not return to baseline. Even on a full rebreather mask, the patient could not converse normally. I took the PCA (patient-controlled analgesic) machine into my office and opened it up to find that the machine had been mistakenly programmed for Morphine instead of Dilaudid—the patient's decreased saturation was a direct result of receiving more than 10 times the normal dose of narcotics.

Just then, the door opened and the nurse who was responsible for the patient came into my office. Before bursting into tears, she mumbled something under her breath. After reviewing the narcotic administration policy and debriefing her shift, I finally asked, "What did you say when you first came into my office? It sounded like 'I shouldn't have let them get to me.'" Immediately the young nurse's eyes shot downward to the floor as she told her story…

> *I was about seven or eight minutes late for my shift last night. When I came around the corner of the nurses' station, a group of nurses who had been talking suddenly stopped when they saw me. I don't mean to be paranoid, but the conversation never picked up again. I went into the ladies room—you can hear from there you know. Ellie said, "She'll never make a good nurse, will she?" Then someone else whose voice I didn't recognize said, "She just doesn't have what it takes. Does she?" I let those words destroy me. This is all my fault.*

No amount of consoling or counseling could remove her pain. Six weeks later she transferred off the unit to the very first open position in the hospital. Was this an isolated event, or a trend? As a manager I realized that if I didn't change the conditions under which this event happened, there was a high possibility it could happen again.

What were those systemic conditions? (Charney and Bartholomew, 2011) There is no doubt that horizontal hostility is deeply institutionalized. When deconstructed, four primary themes of horizontal hostility emerge: economy and workload, lack of interpersonal skills, lack of management skills, and the hierarchical nature of nurses' work (Croft and Cash, 2012). Add to these themes issues such as the mistrust from errors, absent leadership, poor communication skills, and competing values, and a much broader picture emerges. Horizontal hostility is a complex phenomenon—a picture that we can finally see by putting all of these puzzle piece themes together. Deconstructing the causes will then give us the information we need to construct the solutions.

Organizational Context

Hierarchy

Hostility is a natural outcome of working in the hierarchical United States healthcare system, where nurses at the intermediate level have little control and scarce resources. By its very nature, the structure of this system supports oppression. Hierarchy squashes autonomy, diminishes pride and identity, and silences voices.

Nursing can be an autonomous profession (the oxygen rate drops and I can put the patient on oxygen; or I am concerned about a patient's low urine output and increase oral fluid intake [important to change as a nurse can't change the IV], etc.). Yet, as described in earlier chapters, many of the resources nurses need are beyond their control or access. Hierarchical relationships crush autonomy and create a feeling of learned helplessness:

> The patient was going into delirium tremors and another was crawling out of bed but we were not allowed to ask for a sitter, or an extra nursing assistant. There are warning signs plastered all over the place reminding me of patient falls, but I can't catch my patient because I can't be in six rooms at the same time! This was an accident waiting to happen—and it did. And I could not do anything to prevent it.

Just as nurses have been socialized into a culture of learned helplessness with overt and covert clues, so are administrators socialized into their heightened status. Hierarchy is such a defining and pervasive feature of organizations that its forms and basic functions are often taken for granted (Magee and Galinsky, 2008). Status and power hierarchies tend to be self-reinforcing as individuals start thinking and acting in ways that lead to the requisition and acquisition of power. Corporate behaviors that have been a part of the business culture for time immemorial unknowingly support and endorse the power differential:

- Secrecy: meetings are usually held behind closed doors.

- Harm is kept quiet and known by only a few.

- Lack of visibility on front lines sends message that:

  - We have more valuable things to do

  - There is nothing you have that we need to see or hear

  - You are not important

- Lack of transparency around salaries and financials.

  - CEOs make an average of 350 times the salary of employees, which creates resentment

- Lack of approachability—body language is more aloof and less familiar, less eye contact, not knowing your name.

- Feedback, if sought at all, is only solicited from director level.

- Special perks like special parking privileges.

- Performance evaluations are used to socialize and conform.

  - Not weighed on relationships as vital contributions and are not based on an understanding of the role

- Deferring to Human Resources—pulling the "HR card."

  - To have the difficult conversations

- "Us and Them" mentality

- Location of offices—corner offices and views.

  - We eat at a separate dining room

  - We don't socialize together

  - We don't look like you because we dress differently—nicer

  - And have a special exit door for quick exit access

- Lack of trust: promises are broken, e.g., "there will never be any layoffs."

♦ Lack of accessibility: appointments must be made in order to see high-ranking officials, with secretaries as vigilant as if they were guarding famous rock stars.

♦ Positive deviance is frowned upon. If "we" create a new policy, initiative, or practice and you do not agree, then you must not be a team player.

♦ To get promoted, you must imitate and emulate this dominant culture. The game is to get ahead rather than doing the right thing.

These behaviors enable oppression, providing fuel to an already dysfunctional system. Everyone who works in a hospital feels its effects, and, ultimately, so does the patient. The current compressed workload demands that nurses' focus on what is directly in front of them, but what can we learn if we zoom out from the unit where a staff nurse is currently belittling her coworker? This chapter opened with an example of hostility's direct impact on patient care at the bottom of the hierarchy. What does hostility look like in the context of a hospital if we start at the top?

As CEO of a large tertiary hospital, Robert is preparing for his quarterly meeting with the board of directors. He takes a deep breath and stares at the neatly stacked reports piled on his desk. As hospital margins shrink, the cost of doing business rises sharply every year. Medicaid's reimbursement rates are down, the hospital insurance policy deductible has increased 100 fold (from last year's deductible of 1,000 to 100,000), the union is bargaining for higher wages and a better insurance package, and the number of uninsured cases has increased dramatically. Several years ago, Robert eliminated the chief nursing officer and other administrative positions due to advice he had read on hospital restructuring and reorganization in the late 1990s. To make matters worse, patients are now asking for outcomes and satisfaction measurements, and Robert must keep these scores high in order to stay competitive. Frustrated and challenged from all directions, his eyes rivet on the only pile he can control. Robert cuts a half-million dollars from nursing and support services, just as he did last year.

Alex sits at his desk scouring the fourth quarter service excellence reports. As vice president of quality, he is responsible for creating a culture of excellence and does not understand why the numbers haven't changed in almost two years. Even the employee and physician satisfaction scores have not improved significantly, despite a massive campaign to uphold new behavioral standards of customer service. The hospital has invested heavily in consultants to get this project off the ground. Each manager must send thank-you notes to their staff, round with employees, post strategic action plans, and report back—but the numbers just aren't moving. He shoots an urgent email to his director, requesting a meeting.

Eleanor is in charge of the service excellence and service recovery program. She is responsible for compiling all the systemwide reports and presenting them to hospital employees and senior leadership. She has poured a lot of time and energy into making the service excellence program succeed by developing campaigns and presenting at meetings. Two of her employees have been out sick on FMLA (Family Medical Leave of Absence) and, unbeknownst to her, the one remaining employee, Carol, is ready to quit at any minute. Feeling unheard and unsupported, Carol heads to her meeting with Jane, her manager, to resolve a patient complaint—and do some complaining herself.

Jane slams the file cabinet door shut in frustration. For eight years, she has been writing reports, sending emails, and reporting to her boss that she needs more resources to operate the floor, more personnel, and an education space for her elective surgery patients. She has tried to see all 70 patients every week as the service excellence commitments dictate, but that would mean coming in on weekends. Yesterday, she spent almost an hour dealing with an angry patient who did not understand why he didn't routinely receive pain medications every three hours. Another patient's anxiety level was so high that he had a panic attack as soon he hit the floor from surgery. If only they knew what to expect, she wouldn't be spending all her time explaining procedures and protocols to patients who were half-drugged on pain meds anyway! Just then, one of Jane's nurses opens the door with a question on the service excellence report.

"Excuse me," the nurse says. "How many discharge phone calls did we make this month and how many thank-you notes did you write?"

Jane is overwhelmed. She sighs and replies, "Pick a number." The floor is two nurses short for evening shift, and she has already called several nurses, but no one wants to work. Maybe Kim can double?

Kim is clearly irritated by the time the report ends. "I have two amputees and my nursing assistant was late," she complains to the charge nurse.

"Don't worry. I'll help you, and Stephanie's preceptee can help too," the charge nurse replies.

But things just get worse. When Kim asks Stephanie if her preceptee can hang a unit of blood, Stephanie retorts, "She already knows how to do that." Kim is irritated. "Some help," she mutters.

As Kim approaches the main nursing station, she sees that the charge nurse is now making discharge phone calls and is unable to help. Irritated, she turns and barks an order at the nursing assistant who had shown up late.

"Hurry up, the cabulance is coming at 11 and Mr. Walker must be ready!"

The cabulance driver arrives on the floor to pick up Mr. Walker, only to find him in a dirty gown. It's 11:00 a.m., and he has not yet had breakfast. In the commotion that follows as staff race to make last-minute preparations, no one notices that Mr. Walker puts a call in to his friend—on the board of directors.

If any of these "power players" breaks from the current organizational script, then they are immediately marginalized—most commonly by being told that they are "not a team player" or that they are "not a good fit."

Oppression results as the pressures of working in an inefficient and costly system are passed down from one level to another. Oppression is felt in every tier, but its effects are frequently not acknowledged because of intense work demands and the powerful tug of the status quo, and because we are humans who are trying our very best to fit into the "herd." The process and impact of socialization cannot be underestimated. In large organizations, this is frequently the point of disconnect, as staff are so consumed by their individual task and time imperatives that they fail to see the big picture or hear the needs of the subordinate group. It's a one-way conversation: down. As Bruce Avolio, PhD, has observed, information will typically travel no more than two levels below the source.

Lack of Leadership Skills

The fish rots from the head down.
—Old Swedish Proverb

It is well known that the number one reason nurses leave their workplace is because of their relationship with their manager. It is the manager's job to validate and act on the concerns of the staff, to be visible and engaged, to genuinely care for all staff, and to dismantle the hierarchy. But managers often function as a marginalized group because they are stuck in the middle—they do not belong to the dominant *or* oppressed group. And groups that are marginalized typically adopt and align themselves with the behaviors and values of the dominant group in order to survive the corporate culture. Unfortunately, the behaviors and values of the dominant group most closely resemble authoritarian leadership styles and do not lend themselves to leading sustained cultural change.

Leading cultural change requires an authentic transformational leader who ensures that the mission, vision, and values of the organization match the behaviors that they see on their units. The oppressed group values of caring, compassion, and the importance of relationships are vital to cultural transformation. The organizational structure enables the current culture by not setting these clear expectations and/or by not holding leaders accountable.

> *Every nurse had to attend a mandatory in-service on nurse-to-nurse hostility. The chief nursing officer herself gave the introduction for every session and set the expectation that the overt and covert behaviors that were tolerated in the past were "no longer acceptable." But I guess one of her directors was exempt because she continued rolling her eyes and putting down other nurses—so in the end, the CNO's words didn't mean a thing … little changed.*

Historically, charge nurses and managers have been promoted for their clinical skills and frequently lack the interpersonal skills needed to build strong teams (or in my case, because no one else applied for the job). This reflects the values of the dominant group: efficiency, lean, financial. Business savvy has been the most important management skill in the current culture, and staying under budget the most critical factor. Many managers for clinics, ambulatory care centers, and hospitals now no longer need to be nurses. In addition, span of control for many nursing leaders is being threatened. One major consulting company is currently advising hospital executives to have one manager lead three units. Sound familiar?

The slice and dice nursing that occurred in the late 1990s has returned as the Affordable Care Act pushes organizations to change from volume-based to value-based care. Leadership that focuses on creating healthy interdisciplinary teams is clearly vital if we are to redefine the work of nursing and its worth to society.

How the Organizational Structure Enables Oppression

The problem is that hospital restructuring has fundamentally changed the organizational arrangements that shape nurses' daily work lives and what it means to be a nurse.

—*Dana Beth Weinberg*, Code Green

Workload

The increased compression of nurses' work has not been generally acknowledged by industry leaders because nurses have adapted to the increased pace and demand. Human adaptability theory states that changes that are slow and incremental are not noticed by human beings. Over time, the patients are physically heavier and more acute, the patient length of stay has decreased, and time spent charting, the number of drugs available, comorbidities, and diabetes have increased. This overall effect has been coined "compression complexity" (Krichbaum, 2007).

> *I was floated to Oncology and one of my patients had 35 scheduled meds—not PRN! I only knew 17 and desperately tried looking up the other 18 during the shift as I gave them. I cannot honestly say that I knew why all these drugs were given or their side effects. I felt horrible.*

While nursing ratios may have stayed the same for many hospitals, the workload is not the same at all, and the impact of nurse-to-patient ratios must be addressed. In the Aiken study, which examined the link between nurse-to-patient ratio and patient deaths, as well as factors related to RN retention, Aiken and her colleagues found that "higher emotional exhaustion and greater job dissatisfaction were significantly associated with patient-to-nurse ratios." The study linked data from 10,184 staff nurses to 232,342 general, orthopedic, and vascular patients in 1999. For each additional patient over four in a nurse's workload, the risk of death increased by 7% for surgical patients. If the nurse-to-patient ratio was 1:8, patients had a 31% greater risk of dying. "On a national scale, staffing differences of this magnitude may result in as many as 20,000 unnecessary deaths each year" (Aiken et al., 2002). The study also left no doubt that there is a link between staffing levels, burnout, and job satisfaction.

Nurses debate whether staff-patient ratios should be put into place. Some leaders argue that this is not the answer and is counterproductive because the focus should be on patients' acuity and not a number. Others point to the fact that if there isn't a law to protect them, the ratios will be extorted. As a profession, we have become divided and are not asking the right question, which would illuminate the real issue.

The charge nurse is the only person in any organization who is at the point of care and has the most current information about patient acuity and staff nurses' skill and competency. Why is it then that the charge nurse cannot decide the minimal staffing necessary to deliver safe, quality care? Because, historically, they have no authority (power) and the economic survival of any hospital is primarily dependent on finances, so the dominant group controls the "grid." This is a perfect example of oppression at work creating horizontal hostility.

> I had one patient in alcohol withdrawal requiring Lorazepam every hour, one demented patient climbing out of bed, and another on an insulin drip—and we are an orthopedic floor! So I asked the supervisor for an additional aide for night shift, but she said, "Sorry, we need to adhere strictly to the grid. If I gave you an aide then everyone would be asking." After that day, I don't even read the quality propaganda. It's B.S.

> I am a consultant. The hospital was staffing at the 25% level and had seven deaths in the previous year—two of these deaths from falls. So I visited the floor where the patients had fallen: 32 beds and 29 fall precaution signs and 20 turning schedules posted; the ration of nurses to patients was 1:8 on day shift and each nursing assistant had 15 patients. I explained to the board of directors that staffing was the reason these patients died and that more patients would die because what they were expecting was impossible. A year later I discovered that they had changed nothing—said they "couldn't afford it." I wish the "patient experience" included being alive.

Economics

Economics dictate nurse staffing ratios. Healthcare is a $2.9 trillion business because its very existence depends on its ability to be financially viable. Without enough sick people, the current system would collapse. Disease has been profitable for several reasons, and as long as these reasons remain covered, nurses will continue to plug the holes in the dam for as long as they possibly can, often even taking responsibility for system failures that are beyond their control. Expensive, unnecessary, and ineffective treatment is constantly using up the resources we so desperately need to keep our nation healthy. Yet this fact is seldom acknowledged in the current healthcare culture. Nurses are told to cut corners so that their institutions can survive financially. Following the money reveals another story regarding the economics of healthcare, as shown in Figure 5.1.

Many businesses have capitalized on the current healthcare system. It is absolutely vital for all nurses to be aware of the inherent dysfunction of the system in which they work. If not, the human tendency is to believe the story that "we are not good enough" or we can't do it and are therefore inadequate if we can't attain the goals set by the dominant group. Directors and managers especially are caught in a difficult space because they are held responsible for high quality and satisfaction measures yet prevented from access to the resources they need to attain those outcomes.

> *We were told at the capital budget meeting that there would be no capital expenditures approved. But patients constantly complained about my antiquated birthing chair in labor and delivery and I needed a new one. So I put in a requisition for a leg on a new chair—next year I will order another leg, and in about six years, I should have the whole chair!*

> *The lights in the nursery that were keeping the babies warm were not only old, they were the wrong wattage and risked burning the babies. They were actually french-fry warmers, yet I still couldn't get the request approved despite the evidence!*

Add to the typical characteristics inherent in business a growing degree of governmental controls, and the result is rules, regulations, and a rigid system of bureaucratic hierarchy. As we descend the ladder of hierarchy, the pressure (or oppression) increases in intensity for two reasons:

- ◆ First, the lower you go on the food chain, the thicker the veil of oppression. Nurses, who are situated at the *bottom* of the ladder are task-saturated and do not have time for reflective practice which would allow them to address the emotional, social, and physical needs of the unit—especially horizontal hostility. **We can't fight what we can't see. A behavior not named is an invisible dragon.**

- ◆ The second reason that nursing feels such intense oppression is because nurses are feeling the total weight of all the pressures from above. Situated at the bottom of the hierarchical ladder, nursing absorbs the cumulative pressures of

Figure 5.1	Healthcare economics

The high cost of pharmaceuticals: There are over 6,000 drugs. For every one million dollars invested in advertising, the return-on-investment to pharmaceutical companies is 19 million dollars. Only the United States and New Zealand allow TV advertising of pharmaceuticals. Over 200 million dollars was spent by this industry alone for lobbying in 2012.

♦ Gleevec® for leukemia patients costs $90,000/year

♦ Advair® use for 2012 was over 99 million

♦ Pulmicort® costs $175.00 in the U.S. and $20.00 in Britain

♦ BioPharma made a profit of 93 billion dollars in 2011

Income from unnecessary surgeries: Over 300,000 unnecessary operations were performed by ENT surgeons last year on children who did not meet the criteria for surgery as mandated by the ENT surgeons themselves. Over 50% of cardiac stents provide no statistical advantage to lifestyle changes, and over 1.3% of all cardiac procedures are deemed unnecessary when best practice is applied.

Healthcare executive salaries are higher than any other industry: One health group CEO made $102 million in 2009 alone. A recent study in *JAMA Internal Medicine* found that the average nonprofit hospital CEO earned $600,000 annually, although the median compensation was $405,000.

♦ Chargemaster pricing: The cost of supplies, procedures, and tests vary tremendously from one hospital to another. For example, a single box of 4 x 4's for a patient was billed at $77.00 and a plastic wrist immobilizer is $800.00 (*Time*, 2013).

♦ Insurance companies lobby aggressively: U.S. insurance companies spent over $200 billion lobbying against the Affordable Care Act alone in order to be guaranteed access to the 47 million uninsured. Insurance companies charge 17 cents on every dollar.

the organization. The stresses that Robert feels are passed down to Alex, who has his own set of pressures from previous cutbacks and who passes all that down to Eleanor, and so forth. And because nursing is multidisciplinary, it feels pressure from all directions. For example, having no discharge social worker on Saturdays means the nurse must stop and arrange the cabulance; having no nutrition services after 9 p.m. forces the nurse to fix the snacks, etc. Nurses constantly absorb others' work without additional resources and fail to evaluate the effect this has on nursing practice.

To say that the veil of oppression keeps us hidden is extremely accurate: Not only are nurses prevented from seeing clearly out through the veil, but the dominant group cannot see in either. Culture is a powerful potion whose magic is worked upon us all. But all that is needed to take back our power is to see the game.

Interpersonal relationships

Senior administration commonly perceives hostility as a Human Resources challenge, thereby distracting attention away from themselves as the source of the problem and creating an effective buffer and eternal distraction. The prevailing mind-set is that hostility is "a personality or behavioral issue." In truth, "bullying and lateral violence is used as a method of disciplining the workforce to accept the behaviors that maintain the status quo" until it becomes the norm of the work environment (Hutchinson et al., 2010). Surveillance, withholding resources, retaliation, and a host of other tactics constantly ensure that the intangible, invisible, dominant power structure stays in place.

No department is to blame; and no department is exempt. Human Resources does not perceive their enabling role—held captive by a set of archaic practices and intense myopic focus. They are limited of course from changing by the dominant group who keeps all the players in the power game in a checkmate stance. Only compliance is rewarded in the current system, with the status quo assured by managers who are just "doing their job" by imitating the exact same patriarchal tactics they themselves experience. These are learned behaviors, which is why horizontal hostility is so virulent: We are all bullies, victims, and witnesses in the drama, unconsciously and often simultaneously.

Authentic leadership

"...a pattern of leader behavior that draws upon and promotes both positive psychological capacities and a positive ethical climate, to foster greater self-awareness, an internalized moral perspective, balanced processing of information, and relational transparency on the part of leaders with followers, fostering positive self-development"
—Walumbwa et al., 2008, *Journal of Management.*

Administration cannot respond to the needs of a group characterized by silence and invisibility. Nurses immersed in a drama often take negative comments personally and spend their energy licking their own wounds. Alternatively, nurses ignore their wounds because they are too busy or because their primary focus is on the patient. In addition to the general lack of voice, those who do speak are often labeled as being uncooperative and are left feeling unheard and invalidated.

Competing goals: A conflict of interests

The fact that healthcare is a business produces a conflict of interests. Nurses' greatest desire is to provide high-quality care, but although quality is also a goal of the institution, it is not the institution's primary goal. Historically, a hospital's primary goal has been to stay financially viable. This conflict of primary interests produces a profound power struggle and destroys trust because frontline staff can clearly see that administration says one thing and does another.

The pressures passed down by the organization are essentially the result of a struggle for a limited amount of power. In her book *Code Green: Money-Driven Hospitals and the Dismantling of Nursing,* Dana Beth Weinberg discusses power as related to hospital mergers and points out that power is situational (2003). We can view this power in two ways: as a *finite* (limited) amount or an *expanding* amount (Katz and Kahn, 1978). Whether power is finite or expanding depends on whether there is commonality or a conflict of values.

When there are two primary values (i.e., money vs. safe, quality care), power is perceived as finite (Weinberg, 2003). A singular primary vision of patient-centric care is absolutely critical, because this commonality produces a powerful synergy and infinite power. With two competing goals, a struggle for power will always ensue, because power is perceived as finite. This struggle, which administration undeniably wins, leaves nurses feeling powerless.

> *What bothers me the most is that I come with the room charge—like a bed or a water pitcher ... I am insulted because there is nothing that differentiates me from "things."*

Because the general culture operates as if healthcare is a business, nurses are viewed as an interchangeable commodity. "If those who work within the acute healthcare bureaucracy are identified as a commodity rather than a valued asset, there can be a sense of helplessness, lack of autonomy, and perception of no respect arising from a profound feeling of powerlessness" (Sumner and Townsend-Rocchiccioli, 2003).

With the advent of the Affordable Care Act, healthcare in America is literally undergoing a forced revolution. It will no longer be a long-term option for this industry to make money on unnecessary surgeries, patients who have been readmitted, or ineffective, low-quality patient care. The new system, while imperfect in many ways, is no longer willing to pay for our mistakes. Furthermore, the future holds tremendous opportunity for nurses to significantly impact the health of all Americans.

Professional Context

Horizontal hostility not only is inherent in the organizational structure but also stems from conflict within our profession. The most obvious of these conflicts is the profession's lack of consensus concerning the entry-level requirement for nursing: ADN or BSN.

A 2010 Gallup Survey of 1,504 thought leaders across the country found that "thought leaders" from government, corporations, health services, and universities believed nurses had less influence on healthcare reform and its implementation than all other groups, including patients, physicians, insurance companies, pharmaceutical executives, and government. The perception of these leaders was that nurses were not "important decision-makers" and lacked "a single voice."

Perceptions are critical and whether accurate or not must be addressed. It is likely this perception that nurses are poor decision-makers came from the fact that as a profession we cannot decide how many years of college a person should have to be certified as a registered nurse. Despite the research by Aiken and her colleagues that a

10% increase in the proportion of nurses with bachelor's degrees is associated with a 5% decrease in mortality and failure to rescue, the infighting about entry-level college requirements continues (Aiken, 2003). "If we don't stop the infighting, rally around this incredible profession, and form a single powerful governing body representing this workforce of three million strong, we will have failed to rescue ourselves" (Bartholomew, 2010).

Less obvious than this professional discord, however, is the conflict in the very nature of our work itself. In his book *Beyond Caring: Hospitals, Nurses, and the Social Organization of Ethics,* Daniel Chambliss identifies three core features of nurses' work, which he labels "missions" (1996). The nurse is expected, and typically expects herself, to simultaneously be a:

1. Caring individual
2. Professional
3. Relatively subordinate member of the organization

But there is a problem. "The directives conflict: be caring and yet professional; be subordinate and yet responsible, be diffusely accountable for a patient's well-being and yet oriented to the hospital as an economic employer" (Chambliss, 1996).

Weinberg's book *Code Green* gives an important and detailed account of how hospital cost-cutting and downsizing as a response to managed care in the late 1990s magnified this conflict. "In particular, hospital restructuring devalued the caring aspects of nurses' roles, strained their ability to act as professionals, and emphasized their subordination to institutions that find it necessary to emphasize margin over mission" (Weinberg, 2003). Sadly, this pattern repeated itself in 2013 as many hospitals cut their education budgets and systems, and combined resources to form mega-systems as a way to increase purchasing power, cut duplication of services, and ensure viability.

Our fundamental desire to be caring and professional, yet also subordinate, causes a great deal of inner turmoil on a daily basis. Nurses function in a subordinate position with unrealistic institutional expectations. It does not occur to many nurses, especially nurse managers, that what is being asked of them is unreasonable. We spend a lot of wasted energy trying to get the resources we need to do our jobs. We are expected to continuously provide a certain standard of care—indeed "ordered to care in a society that refuses to value caring" (Reverby, 1987).

Caring is one of the fundamental tenets of nursing. By caring, we create and hold a space so that our patients can heal. As much as it is physical, and is surely intellectual, nursing is emotional work. When our hearts are wounded, the care we deliver is far from optimal. If we are upset, we can't think straight. No nurse, especially those at the first line of defense—the bedside—can afford for this to happen. The mental and emotional state of nurses is a critical human factor. There is an obvious and direct link between our emotions and our mental clarity—and our mental clarity and patient safety.

First do no harm?

Another undercurrent that travels just below the radar is the belief that a good physician or nurse does not make mistakes—that being human is akin to perfection. This cultural meme begins in school and destroys the foundation of trust that our patients have in us and that we have in each other.

When I spoke last year to a group of third-year medical students on the topic of creating a just culture, I asked, "When was the last time you did something wrong?" A voice from the back of the room called out, "When was the last time I did anything right?" These medical students felt belittled for being human. It is no wonder then that we have a culture where it is a professional stigma to make a mistake. Because of this dysfunctional belief, we tend not to share our near-misses that others could learn from—and we hide the harm itself.

When harm is not visible, a culture of mistrust and fear prevails and the tendency is to blame the last person who touched the patient. Blame is "a way to discharge fear and pain" (Brown, 2010). In a tragic sequence of events on September 19, 2010, a 9-month old infant died in part as a result of a miscalculated medication dose, and seven months later the critical care nurse who administered that medication committed suicide (Charney, 2011).

It is absolutely critical that nurses support each other from frontline staff to managers and boards of nursing. If we do not create a culture where we know that we have "each other's backs" and feel protected, then fear will continue to pull us apart.

Making all harm visible is the first step. At Cincinnati Children's Hospital, for example, a message appears on the home screen which answers the question, "How many days since a child has been harmed in our care?" thus engaging employees in every department to learn more about how their particular roles can keep patients safe.

Don Berwick, MD, MPP, cofounder of the Institute for Healthcare Improvement (IHI) in Boston, is well known for saying, "Every system is perfectly designed to produce the results it consistently achieves." This statement was first applied in the automobile industry to illustrate that car quality was a direct result of the factory process. We know the results in healthcare:

- Serious harm seems to be 10–20 times more common than lethal harm
- Lethal harm is estimated at over 400,000 preventable deaths per year (James, 2013)
- Nurses are dissatisfied and leaving while we face the worst nursing shortage in history, and while we deal with having an inadequate number of faculty

No one disagrees that the system is broken and not working.

- We spend almost twice as much as every other industrialized nation ($9,200 per capita) with relatively weak quality metrics to show. The U.S. is 37th in overall health, 39th in infant mortality, 36th in life expectancy, etc.
- Healthcare costs are unevenly distributed. Only 1% of the population spends 35% of all healthcare dollars. And just 5% of the population of the United States uses over 60% of our healthcare resources.
- We tolerate an unacceptable variation in quality, safety, service, and cost (up to 1000%). For example, a total knee can cost $14,000–51,000. The exact same ankle surgery is $200,000 in New York and $40,000 in New Hampshire. Where you live determines what surgery you are most likely to get (See the Dartmouth Atlas at *www.dartmouthatlas.org/*).

Yet despite these well-known facts, the public is not up in arms. And although nurses constitute a significant enough percentage of the population to take a strong stand themselves, nurses have not united to address the problem. Horizontal hostility is a critical impediment to solidarity. It is the antithesis of teamwork. Nurses are not speaking out in one unified voice to change the system, but they could. Until we begin to listen and make our voices heard, it will be impossible to unite to address the bigger issues.

The Role of Unions

We fear things in proportion to our ignorance of them.

—*Christian Nestell Bovee*

If solidarity is critical for nurses to effect any significant change in American health-care, are unions the answer? There is absolutely no debating the important role that unions have played in providing increased wages and benefits for nurses over the last few decades, as well as basic human rights like maternity leave. Nurses joined unions so that they would have more bargaining power because an individual nurse's voice was about as effective as whispering from the nosebleed section of a ballpark. When nurses banded together and unionized, they felt more powerful because, finally, they were heard.

This question can only be answered by unions themselves: What is the primary goal of the union? Is it to elevate nurses to a point where union power is not as necessary because nurses have taken back their own voices and power? Or is it to fight for and protect nurses? If the goal is to elevate the voice and power of nurses, then there will be a day in the far future when unions have successfully accomplished this goal and nurses are esteemed and valued by society. If the goal is to be the defender, then those we shield may eventually fall into the trap of perceiving themselves as a vulnerable population. The caution is to always be aware that there can only be one primary goal.

All nurses must unite: union and non-union, ADN and BS, frontline and senior leaders. Until then, we are still divided. Unions are perfectly positioned to provide education that challenges the current paradigm. They have a tremendous opportunity to elevate nurses' self-esteem, increasing the personal and professional power of nurses by providing education on assertive communication skills, and emphasizing the tremendous contribution that nurses make to their patients and society. Herein lies an opportunity for all of us to work together with an energy born of our collective passion: to heal humanity.

Emotional state

In her book *Transforming Nurses' Stress and Anger: Steps Toward Healing*, Sandra Thomas summarizes the themes that emerged from years of gathering nurses' stories about their stress and anger:

◆ "I feel overloaded and overwhelmed."

◆ "I am not treated with respect."

◆ "I am blamed and scapegoated."

◆ "I feel powerless."

◆ "I am not being heard."

◆ "I feel morally sick."

◆ "I am not getting any support."

The powerlessness and helplessness expressed in these statements is overwhelming. But these are not the only stressors nurses feel. If we expand our focus to include the daily challenges of living in the present day in the United States, it is easy to see why "everyday nursing" can feel like an emotional percolator.

In the Context of Our World

I have always considered myself the queen of multitasking—the divine diva of efficiency. So last summer, I had carefully calculated that I had just enough time before my 2:00 p.m. meeting to take my son to the doctor. He had injured his shoulder in the spring, and months later it was still hurting. As I got into the car at the parking garage, I saw the yellow sticky note I had carefully placed on the dashboard earlier that day that read, "Don't forget the x-rays." No problem, I thought. Last night I had done a visual check and they were behind the bookcase.

Everything was running smoothly until the moment the doctor held up the x-rays to the light. At first he scrunched up his face. Then, with a straight face, he turned to me and said, "Mrs. Bartholomew, I have some bad news. Your son is a small dog."

In my haste and efficiency, I had grabbed the dog's x-rays instead of my son's.

No one comes to work and leaves all of their problems at home. We can't swipe in our badges and simultaneously wipe out our minds, deleting all the things we worry about outside of work. Nurses, as well as other professionals, bring their problems with them to the workplace.

"The year 2000 marked the first time that less than a quarter (23.5%) of American households were made up of a married man and woman and one or more children—a drop from 45% in 1960. The number is expected to fall to 20% by 2010" (Sado and Bayer, 2001). These numbers mean that nurses are often single parents who carry additional responsibilities that add additional stressors to everyday life. Phone calls interrupt a nurse's daily routine as she tries to figure out who can pick Johnny up from school and then who will take care of him until she gets home.

Additionally, for the first time in history, our children are sicker than their parents (McDonough, 2002). The largest growing segment of the population for prescription drugs is children under the age of 19—despite the fact that the 65+ generation has grown by 10% (Putnam, 2000). Some of the major problems these drugs are addressing in young people are hyperactivity, depression, high blood pressure, and diabetes.

When I hurt myself at work, to tell you the truth, it was a relief. I had to stay home for three weeks. I got to stop. I got to remember what "stop" was.

Furthermore, membership in both professional and recreational groups has decreased significantly in the last 50 years (Putnam, 2000). We are simply too busy for it. As a result, our social support group is faltering, and we are becoming more isolated. Social skills normally practiced in group settings are declining. The pressures of our life mount with the realization that we are "on our own."

One of the most important indicators of intent to stay is a sense of belonging. How important is belonging? "Joining any group at all cuts in half your chances of dying" (Putnam, 2000). But you can't belong to a group if no one knows you, if no one ever has any downtime, or if the pace of work is so intense you can't get a break or eat lunch. Yet the majority of us spend more time with our coworkers in any given week than we do with our families.

If I do get a break, I use that time to make appointments for car repairs or doctor visits for the kids. When I ride the ferry to work, I use that time to pay my bills.

In 1965, economists predicted that in the year 2000, Americans would have more than 600 billion hours of additional leisure time due to all of the time-saving inventions of that period. How are we spending our time? Instead of vacationing, we now work 60+ hours a week and 61% of us work when we are supposed to be on vacation. For the first time in history the rich work longer hours than the poor because of their access to technology. Our "speed dialing, speed dating, fast track, express line, quickie mart" life is taking its toll.

Nurses feel the stressors of their organization, their profession, and their world—and don't always deal with them in a healthy manner. The American Nurses Association (ANA) estimates that 6%–8% of nurses use alcohol or other drugs to the extent that they impair their professional performance.

The average age of a nurse (48 years) has risen sharply over the past few years, primarily due to the nursing shortage. Most of these nurses have a career of 25 or more years, and the physical and mental wear and tear on their bodies has had a cumulative effect. Nurses are experiencing injuries that they are not reporting to their hospitals due to labor-intensive paperwork and the inability to find a physician who accepts labor and industry compensation. Once again, administration cannot address a problem it does not know exists.

Food for Thought: Exercises

1. Explain why the pull to maintain the status quo is so powerful in institutions.

2. Identify three behaviors used by the dominant group in your workplace to ensure the power equilibrium and describe the effect of these behaviors.

3. Read "Deconstructing bullying and lateral violence" *(www.ncbi.nlm.nih.gov/pubmed/23181374)*. Choose one of the four prisms of understanding and either concur or argue validity from your work experience point of view.

4. In your experience, do you think horizontal hostility exists among nurse practitioners? Why or why not?

5. Imagine that in 2014, nurses come together as a group and decide the entry level into the profession is a bachelor's degree, and a master's degree within five years. Fast-forward 30 years. What impact might this have on the future of nursing? Describe this vision.

6. Read the quote below. Could expecting hospitals to provide health benefits actually be helping them maintain their dominant or patriarchal role?

> *...employers in the long run should not provide healthcare insurance. In a world where my son will have 9–12 jobs by the time he is 35 it is insane to have employers play that role. In the long run it would be a lot better for all those employers to put their workers in the exchange.*
>
> —Andy Stern, Seattle Town Hall, January 7, 2013

Summary

Viewing hostility in the context of the organization, our profession, and our world gives us some additional clues about why horizontal hostility occurs. In our current healthcare system, nurses suffer from a profound sense of powerlessness, a lack of autonomy, decreased job satisfaction and morale, and a weak identity. These characteristics are all associated with oppressed groups.

From applying the oppression theory, we know that:

♦ Infighting is a known attribute of any oppressed group

♦ Attributes originally valued by the subordinate group are devalued

♦ This devaluation manifests itself in low self-esteem

From studying animals, we know that:

♦ Primates are known for displacing aggression

♦ Three factors increase psychological stress

  – The lack of an outlet for frustration

  – The lack of social support systems

  – Unpredictability

From an organizational and professional context, we know horizontal hostility emerges due to:

♦ A lack of voice or representation in the organization's hierarchical structure

♦ A conflict of primary interests with the dominant group

- A constant power struggle for finite resources

- Increasing pressure on hospitals to survive financially (which is heavily felt on the bottom tier—nursing)

- A lack of solidarity within our own profession, which prevents mobilization of resources

From the context of the world we live in, we know that:

- Nurses face mounting pressures in their personal lives

- There has been a significant decrease in social support networks

- Staff bring outside pressures to the workplace

Resources

Overtreated by Shannon Brownlee

Code Green: Money-Driven Hospitals and the Dismantling of Nursing by Dana Beth Weinberg

Nursing Against the Odds: How Healthcare Cost-Cutting, Media Stereotypes, and Medical Hubris Undermine Nurses and Patient Care by Suzanne Gordon

Transforming Nurses' Stress and Anger: Steps Toward Healing by Sandra P. Thomas

The Healing of America by T.R. Reid

Section 2

Best Practices to Eliminate Horizontal Hostility

Section 2

Best Practices to Eliminate Horizontal Hostility

Introduction

*I remain convinced that a transformation must take place in nursing,
a transformation in the hearts and minds of individual nurses that ultimately
creates peace and harmony in our relationships with one
another. If we do not link arms to face today's formidable challenges,
nursing's future could be in jeopardy.*

—*Sandra Thomas*

The question is: how do we change course? Given the increasing pressures on everyone in nursing, from university professors to student nurses, it seems that our energy can best be spent in a unified, passionate, and immediate response. Understanding the forces that contribute to horizontal hostility (Section I) was the first step. Taking action is the second (Section II).

Just as Section I gave us a conceptual framework for understanding horizontal hostility, Section II provides us with a conceptual framework for the solution. **Our solution lies in the etiology, or study of causation, of the problem.** Therefore, we must recognize that:

- Because hierarchy diminishes two-way communication and power, **leveling the playing field will decrease hostility**

- Because powerlessness is a result of an unequal, finite amount of power, **empowering nurses and encouraging voice will decrease hostility**

- Because silence and closed systems perpetuate horizontal hostility, **creating an environment where staff feel free to communicate (to speak their truth) is critical, as is changing to an open system**

- Because horizontal hostility is insidious, **bringing the subject out into the open will decrease its prevalence**

- Because decreased self-esteem is a common theme in oppressed groups (and because it maintains the status quo), **any intervention directed at increasing esteem will decrease horizontal hostility**

- Because pressure has increased in the workplace and we have adapted to a great deal of unconscious stressors, **stopping to acknowledge these pressures will increase awareness and decrease frustration/hostility**

- Because a faster pace of work does not allow us time to see the consequences of our actions, **reflective practice will allow us an opportunity to see how our behaviors affect each other and decrease hostility**

- Because a belief system of subordination accompanies oppression, **illuminating these beliefs and creating a new archetype will foster healthy work attitudes**

- Because the lack of a social support network increases aggression, **increasing social support networks will decrease psychological stress**

The following chapters contain specific examples and interventions for building a healthy work culture and decreasing horizontal hostility. The common denominator in all of these interventions will be:

- Leveling the playing field (i.e., decreasing stratification)
- Empowering staff by increasing voice or agency
- Raising awareness
- Increasing self-esteem
- Creating an open communication network
- Providing opportunities for reflection
- Increasing social support networks
- Illuminating the problem by bringing the consequences into the open

We can only take action to the extent that we can distance ourselves from the problem. This distance from the drama, or the emotional issues of our workplace, gives us a new perspective empowered with solutions. As leaders, we are keenly aware of the pressures of working in healthcare, but we are extremely engaged in day-to-day operations. To heal horizontal hostility, we need to step out of this world.

The Big Picture: An Analogy

Actors: Our feelings; **acting out** the hostile behavior

Audience: The part of ourselves that **reflects** on our actions

Director: Our thinking self; the part of ourselves that **critically analyzes** and has the ability to delete, add lines, or write a new script

The Scene: Think of a large opera house. In the Opera House are many theaters, and in each theater a play is **NOW SHOWING!**

In theater number one, *Horizontal Hostility* is playing. This drama began decades ago as a one-act play called *Join Us If You Can*, featuring new nurses being educated into the hospital setting. Nobody remembers who wrote that script—probably because it was a doctor.

About ten years ago, the play became a full-length feature portraying the intense drama in the relationships among nurses and was renamed *Horizontal Hostility.* You have to be really smart to get a role in this play—and have a very large bladder capacity, because there are no bathroom breaks. If you can find the time to eat something, you won't remember what you ate because you are too busy concentrating on juggling your responsibilities.

All the actors are playing nurses. Some actors have main roles, some play supporting roles, and some you can't distinguish from the scenery. Nurses learn their lines as understudies, so the nonstop acting has been able to run continuously for years. This is primarily because when you have a play going 24 hours a day, you can't stop the momentum. Like a merry-go-round that's always spinning, actors learn how to jump on and off on cue.

There is no audience. After you play a role for 40,000 or so hours, like most of the crew, you forget about the audience because the play itself requires so much energy.

In theater number two, *A Day in the Life of a Manager* is playing. New actresses for this role are just thrown on stage and learn by improvising. Usually, you can get a job here very easily because there is never a waiting list. The action is intense—stand-up tragedy. When the play was popular 20 years ago, some of the managers could take a break and go see *Horizontal Hostility,* but that hasn't happened for a long time.

No one can remember an audience. It's even hard for the managers to remember where they parked their cars because it's usually dark out when they start and dark again when they go home. If you miss your cue (or just admit that you can never find your car), you lose your role. Most people think that's a bad thing.

In theater numbers three and four are the directors and administrators—all very involved in their own dramas, but with a *much bigger orchestra.* There are no props, and the scenery is bleak. They can't miss a beat and the music never stops. It is virtually impossible for anyone to step out of their role or they might miss some critical dialogue in the play, so nobody has left the stage for a long time. They don't break to eat, nor do they show any emotion, which has led some outsiders to wonder if they are even human.

In the last theater is the CEO. He's doing a soliloquy—available on DVD.

From the audience, the impact of horizontal hostility is clear. Stepping out of the play and into the audience is the only way we can understand the drama. Only from this perspective can we reflect on our actions. This is how we illuminate the behavior. By doing so, we see that there is indeed a larger setting. We can anticipate the next scene and realize the effect horizontal hostility has on all the characters—pain.

If we can simply step out of the drama long enough to find the director—that part of ourselves that can write a new script—we can end the cycle of hostility.

> **Every day,**
> **in every interaction,**
> **we either approve of the old script**
> **or write a new one.**

C h a p t e r   6

Nurturing Our Young

The importance of RNs is expected to increase in the coming decades, as new models of care delivery, global payment, and a greater emphasis on prevention are embraced ... will the nursing workforce be ready to respond to these challenges?

—*Auerbach et al.*, New England Journal of Medicine (2013)

Learning Objectives

1. List two impediments to a healthy student or resident nurse experience.

2. Compose a plan for a successful new hire experience in your workplace.

It is time to build a new archetype: an ideal of nursing whose belief system empowers nurses and recognizes the unique and critical role they play in our society. A logical place to start is with the new generation of nurses. Our sincere gratitude for choosing nursing must become the hallmark of our mentoring.

Of critical importance in the nursing shortage is the fact that "60% of newly registered nurses leave their first position within six months because of some form of lateral violence perpetrated against them" (Griffin, 2004). Researchers in New Zealand found that horizontal hostility was a common experience for first-year nurses and that half of the horizontal hostility new graduates experienced was not reported. In addition, researchers found that these new nurses lacked the skills needed to deal with hostility (McKenna et al., 2003).

Not only do new nurses experience hostility, but the prevalence increases every year: 18% in the first year, 33% in the second, and 46% in the third year (Cho et al., 2012). This is a clear indication that new nurses are being assimilated into a culture that tolerates negative overt and covert behaviors and lack the interpersonal skill set to effectively end horizontal hostility.

> *My orientation was spent crying in the bathroom. The strange part was that no one did anything about the behavior. The manager felt that we had a communication problem and that we didn't understand each other—a personality conflict.*

> *Everything about [the ICU nurse's] tone was condescending. The message was loud and clear, but unspoken. She was precepting a new nurse, and as soon as she saw me she started putting me down, as if to make it clear that there was a hierarchy even within nursing—that an ICU nurse was much more important than a floor nurse.*

Impediments to a Healthy New Nurse Experience

Staff workload

Downsizing in hospitals has forced employees to take on multiple new tasks, often with a decrease in available resources and an increase in job complexity (Keuter et al., 2000). The result is an increased workload. "Experienced nurses who are already working in stressful conditions with continuous staff shortages and poor recognition of service see the student nurse sometimes as an extra hindrance to their already increasing workload" (Davey, 2002). As pointed out earlier, the work of nursing has become increasingly more complex and compressed.

> *Due to the grid, when I am precepting a new nurse, I still have the same number of patients that I do every other day. It's ridiculous. If someone just followed me for a day, they would see that I can't give these new nurses the attention they deserve.*

Over the years, experienced nurses have picked up new ways of coping with the stress of their workload. I inadvertently discovered one of these innovative approaches one day when I met with a student nurse and a preceptor to find out more details about a medication error that had occurred. The student had given the wrong medication to the wrong patient and the instructor had called me, alarmed. As it turned out, the precepting nurse had taught the student her shortcut: She was pulling out pills before they were due on a patient and keeping them in her pocket. But that was not the only example of nurses trying to cope with the time crunch:

> *The night nurse was complaining vehemently when I entered the ward about the inconvenience of the new medication bar coding system. I approached her and asked, "What's your work-around?"*
>
> *At first, she responded, "I don't know what you mean." But immediately I replied, "I'm a nurse. What's your work-around?" Slowly she pushed up her sleeve to reveal eight patient armbands preprinted on her wrist.*

Erroneous assumptions

Every day in nursing brings incremental pressures that were not there the day before: escalating acuity, physically heavier patients, shorter lengths of stay, new technology and treatments, and higher staff ratios. Advances in technology and pharmacology have resulted in an increase in pills and information that challenges even experienced nurses. Therefore, from a clinical standpoint, new resident nurses are never walking into the same scenario as their mentors.

One would think that experienced nurses would welcome new grads in a nursing shortage. Last year, I decided to put a new resident nurse into the hands of one of our younger nurses who had been with us for five years. Her lack of patience and harsh expectations took me by surprise. After speaking to the nurse, I learned her underlying belief system: "If I did it, she can too. If I had to do orientation in 12 weeks, so should she." This could be considered a hazing or induction phase, which is also commonly practiced among physicians. In every comment, the nurse was comparing the new resident nurse to herself and to her own experience. Experienced nurses feel justified treating new grads harshly because they do not trust their competency (Walrath, Dang, and Nyberg, 2010).

Beliefs drive our behaviors. And the belief system that must be illuminated and challenged is *If I had to prove myself to become a good nurse, then you have to too.*

Traditionally held beliefs about nurses

One hundred nurses in a small community hospital were asked: What is a good nurse?

- A good nurse values him/herself last
- A good nurse completes everything and charts correctly—whether reasonable or not
- A good nurse picks up extra shifts
- A good nurse doesn't leave any task undone
- A good nurse never makes a mistake
- A good nurse doesn't rock the boat
- If I had to earn it, then you will have to as well

Challenging beliefs and our basic assumptions about what makes a good nurse must start in nursing school. Since our beliefs drive our everyday behaviors, it is up to nursing leaders to require nurses to articulate these long-standing cultural memes. For example, as a high-reliability organization, healthcare can only safely be delivered by teams of professionals that communicate seamlessly with each other. The belief that "A good nurse does not need the help of others" is the antithesis of teamwork and sets new nurses up for failure from the start. A preceptor can easily reinforce this belief with an offhand comment of, "You mean you didn't finish the patient's dressing change yet?" The everyday conversations held by faculty, managers, staff nurses, and preceptors continually reinforce our belief system—and vice versa.

Evolutionary new beliefs about nurses

- A good nurse takes care of him/herself
- A good nurse needs the help and support of his/her peers
- A good nurse seizes the details of a mistake and shares them to improve practice
- A good nurse speaks his/her truth at all times
- A good nurse nurtures and feeds new nurses
- A good nurse demonstrates professionalism at all times
- A good nurse constantly prioritizes and may not always finish their work

New nurse perceptions

The profession of nursing has an obligation to reduce lateral violence. The population of newly registered nurses is an ideal place to start. They collectively represent the profession of the future.

—Griffin (2004)

Studies show that the number one clinical teaching behavior that students seek in their instructors is approachability, followed by fairness, openness, honesty, and mutual respect (Viverais-Dresler and Kutschke, 2001). Yet as the pace of work on the floor increases, nurses and preceptors become less approachable than ever—and difficult to connect with because they don't slow down. Time to bond has decreased as nurses skip meals and social interaction dwindles due to 12-hour shifts.

Lacking an understanding of the pace of the floor and the intensity of the workload, new nurses believe that they are in the way, which often leads to feelings of rejection and a lack of the bonding that is so critical to new grads. In addition, the whining and complaining new nurses hear from others causes them to question their choice of nursing as a career.

Almost every clinical experience when I walk up to the nurses' station looking for a nurse to partner with for the day, I get a disgusted, eye-rolling look in return.

I needed to give an update on the patient's status. The nurse didn't have time to discuss it with me. Student nurses to her were a bother and an encumbrance.

What defines a successful shift to a new grad? As the number of tasks and complexity of patients increased, the focus changed from the "plan of care" to the "plan to get out of here on time." Overtime is frowned upon by management in a system where financials are paramount. So the focus of new nurses becomes medication delivery, charting, and clinical interventions—anything that must be charted. And the therapeutic relationship, which cannot be quantified or charted, is not perceived to be worth as much as the clinical tasks, primarily because no one asks for this information.

In summary, the feelings that student and new-to-practice nurses experience the most frequently are that they are an *imposition*, a nuisance, or added work to a group of nurses who are already task-saturated. A content analysis of stories written by junior nurses described four levels of injustice student nurses experience:

- "We were unwanted and ignored"
- "Our assessments were distrusted and disbelieved"
- "We were unfairly blamed"
- "I was publicly humiliated" (Thomas and Burk, 2009)

In a recent survey, dozens of nurses relayed stories reflecting a lack of support, attention, and time as they struggled to complete their assignments (Bartholomew, 2012), and unfortunately, some of these stories included nursing faculty.

Shining a Light on Horizontal Hostility in Nursing Schools

To be vulnerable is to be susceptible to being wounded or hurt, or open to moral attack or criticism ... nursing faculty are seldom viewed as a vulnerable population ... yet they are.

—DalPexxo and Jett (2008)

To say that horizontal hostility started in nursing school—or in any one arena, for that matter—would be to deny its cyclical nature. It started long ago in the subordinate origins of nursing, gathered momentum with a host of factors discussed in Section I, and now permeates every level of our profession. Because it is a part of the culture, no one in nursing is immune to its effects.

Every profession has a particular culture that is reinforced in school by its educators. If we are to change the culture, educators must be aware of and discuss the overt and covert ways that we disempower other nurses. "Students are not encouraged from the start. There is more emphasis on judging than on assisting and supporting them" (Thomas, 2004). Entry-level requirements are so high that classes are filled primarily with highly competitive Type A personalities. Looking back in time reveals how a tough, judgmental culture could have evolved.

My aunt graduated from her nursing program in 1956—the year I was born. Over half of her class was dropped before graduation because her professors were instructed to "weed out the weak ones." The rationale for this approach was that some nurses could not survive the hard physical and emotional work or be able to hold their own with the physicians, many of which had strong personalities. Nurses were to stand up when a physician entered the ward and the pecking order was extremely clear. Both medical and nursing education was patterned after the military (discharge orders, pinning ceremony, uniforms, symbols, etc.) Probation was set at nine months to ensure that the graduates were not pregnant. Today, more than a half century later, the belief that we must be harsh to produce a good nurse—or treat others as we were taught—still prevails as one of our cultural memes.

When I graduated with my masters in nursing I was offered a tenure-track position at a local nursing college. But the salary offered for this full-time position was exactly half of my current salary—$47,000 instead of $95,000. With five children to support, I couldn't accept no matter how much I loved to teach. But it was impossible not to notice the broader cultural discrepancy. The nursing building was shared with the business school whose graduates would all start at over $100,000 when they graduated with a master's degree. In the hierarchy of departments at any university, nursing reflects the greater values of society where science, sports, and technology trump art and the humanities (the football coach receives $8 million, and the professor $84,000.)

It is my observation that of all nursing groups, nursing faculty are the most oppressed. The more oppression, the less the chance that anyone in the group can see the horizontal hostility caused by domination. Salaries for this group are lower than most hospital nurses, and they are "susceptible to physical, psychological, and emotional harm from students, peers, and administrators" (DalPezzo and Jett, 2008). Uncivil encounters with students are usually less severe; however, research shows that subtle interactions have a cumulatively greater impact on stress than life-threatening events. The epitome of potential harm of course occurred in 2002 when three nursing professors were specifically targeted and killed by a student in Arizona who was failing.

Heavy workloads, lack of resources, low morale, abuse and unrealistic expectations from administration, sparse clinical rotations, rude and entitled student behavior, and a general lack of respect have taken their toll on many faculty as they struggle to keep their passion and dedication to teaching alive. Even within the nursing profession, there is a derogatory phrase that many professors have shared which sums up the perception of their worth from other nurses: *"If you can't nurse, teach."* This is a perfect example of horizontal hostility.

When humans are overpowered day in and day out, they then unconsciously release the energy that cannot be directed upward toward each other, and sometimes, toward those with even less power than themselves. (The reason that students are not the most oppressed is because they have an exit plan; by the nature of the program, they will be leaving. Psychologically, when you are in a situation with no foreseeable exit, oppression is intensified.)

> *I was doing a med-pass and had forgotten to check the status of the current IV. My instructor made a "teaching moment" of it during clinical conference and the way he imitated me—his tone and facial expression—made me sound and look like an idiot.*

Characteristics of horizontal hostility among nursing faculty

- Setting up
- Distorting
- Misrepresenting and lying
- Shaming, betraying
- Breaking boundaries
- Splitting, mandating, blaming, and silencing (Heinrich, 2007)

Supporting our faculty

The most frequent forms of horizontal hostility experienced by nursing faculty are ostracism, blaming, competitiveness, bullying, silencing, lack of recognition, devaluation of accomplishments, and a lack of support (Glass, 2003, 2007; Heinrich, 2007). Abuse from administration most commonly takes the form of a profound lack of resources for the Colleges of Nursing.

Last year when I visited a university, I noticed that the nursing office was extremely small, cramped with furniture, and in the basement. After a meeting with the assistant dean, I learned that a team of consultants had been brought in to identify new ways of cutting corners because "our budget has been decreased by 10 million."

The dean's office was already a closet, and so I suggested, "Why don't you tell them that you can't do it?" But as in every case of power imbalance, the oppression is not seen by the powerless group because the dominant group infers that you are "not a team player" and has historically fired anyone who could not play the game.

No is the only word an oppressed group can never say.

Although I was the one who presented the new curriculum idea, no one said anything when another professor acted like it was her idea all along. I sat in the faculty meeting stunned, looking around for validation ... but no one would even make eye contact with me ... I began to doubt myself.

Strategies to minimize peer hostility among faculty are geared toward changing the overall culture and follow the same guidelines for any organization:

1. Start at the top with the leaders setting clear expectations
2. Demonstrate the impact
3. Solicit feedback
4. Raise awareness and skills
5. Establish a new set of norms for dealing with interpersonal conflict

The faculty shortage is much more critical than the nursing shortage; educators are the lifeline of our profession. Strengthening the teaching environment and building a supportive education culture will reap exponential benefits that ripple throughout the entire nursing culture.

My instructor was so wonderful the way she let me try three times to get the IV started and then said, "That was the most difficult stick I've ever seen. You were great." I felt so empowered ... that was the moment I believed that I could really be a great nurse.

There were 18 of us that graduated from the second degree program last year. My orientation to the cardiac unit was wonderful! Everyone was so supportive and encouraging—but that was not what I heard from my classmates. Some of them didn't fare as well as I did ... and are just toughing it out.

Supporting our students

Consider using these strategies to create a supportive atmosphere for nursing students:

1.   **Establish a relationship and expectations.** A good relationship with the manager or charge nurse on the unit helps establish a good student experience. Therefore, when a new group of student nurses comes to the floor, have one consistent contact meet and welcome them as a group. Take this opportunity to communicate these expectations:

     – Students will have a valuable and positive experience

     – Any problems will be brought to the manager's attention

     – The manager's door is open for feedback

     – Students are valued and honored, and feedback will be sought

There have been times on our unit when students clearly felt like they were an imposition and a hindrance to their mentors. Counseling the mentors helped improve the situation tremendously. Caught in the momentum of their work, preceptors were not aware that they were coming across as unavailable and unappreciative. This would have never been discovered without making clear the importance of having an open door policy, establishing a relationship, and soliciting feedback.

2.   **Educate the students.** As the first group of students rotated through our unit, complaints from members of the nursing staff started piling up. The majority were territorial: "They're in our space," "I can't tape report when they're in there at 2:00," "They interrupt me to ask where another nurse is," etc.

To deal with the issue, the charge nurses got together to problem solve. They produced a one-page sheet for the students, called "Tips for a Great Nursing Experience." The sheet began with a sincere welcome: "We are very excited to have students on our unit and want to work together to make it a positive experience for all." It ended with, "We hope your experience was valuable. Please feel free to let us know how we can best work with you. We would love to hear your feedback."

Tips included the following:

     – Please vacate the conference room a half hour before end of shift so nurses can tape report.

- Try to avoid change of shift for data collection.

- Ask the charge nurse for help if your nurse is busy (rather than asking other nurses).

- Give all new orders to the unit secretary promptly. Notify your nurse immediately of any urgent or stat orders.

Instructors provided students with the tip sheet upon arrival, and we never heard another complaint.

> **Tip**   Ask students and nurses to make up a tip sheet for your unit.

3. **Educate all staff nurses.** At staff meetings, I point out emphatically that students and new grads are not walking into the same world that current nurses found when they started. We need to demonstrate this fact to all parties involved and make sure that they understand and acknowledge this difference. Changes that are slow and incremental often go unnoticed, as explained by the human adaptability theory presented in Chapter 2 (in short: "incremental increases in pressure over time go unrecognized and allow pressure to build up without notice"). Here are a few simple examples I use for teaching:

   - *The telephone.* Remember when you would let the telephone ring seven or eight times before hanging up? It was less than 10 years ago, but now that number has slowly gone down to three or four rings—or tweeting 140 characters! Changes that are not noticeable and that happen over time are not obvious.

   - *The frog parable.* If you put a frog into hot water, he jumps out immediately. If you put a frog into cool water and slowly turn up the temperature, the frog will boil to death. At no point will he jump out. How hot is the water at your facility? The temperature of the water that new grads are jumping into today is much hotter than it used to be.

   - *Nursing.* Over the past 10 years, there have been numerous incremental changes in the nurses' workload on the unit. There are many more drugs available, more patients with secondary and chronic illness, an increasingly obese patient population, and a decreasing length of stay.

The result of sharing this perspective has been an increase in compassion and understanding, with staff nurses reframing their attitudes and demonstrating more empathy. New nurses feel less judged and feel validated for the difficulties they are experiencing and report feeling a greater level of support.

4.   **Hold an annual roundtable with the managers from the hospital and instructors that have clinical rotations.** At one of our roundtable discussions, we learned that students reported not feeling like the institution went out of its way for students. An all-day event, scheduled to kick off the year, remedied the problem. With nurses scattered throughout the hospital, an event that brings all parties together for the purpose of validating, connecting, and imparting the values of that institution is prudent. It is an opportunity for CNOs and nursing leadership to increase their visibility and for managers to showcase their own departments.

5.   **Revise the curriculum.** Education must address the culture and social construct of nursing. There should not be any surprises when new nurses hit the floor. Asking nurses to transition from school to the real world without preparing them is a setup for failure. (It's like learning the facts of life—very helpful before your first date.) An in-depth understanding of horizontal hostility will enable students not only to handle difficult situations but also to be catalysts for change. High-level communication and assertiveness skills should be taught and practiced. If these new skills are not rehearsed, then they will not be used. "Providing an educational forum on lateral violence for newly licensed nurses in orientation is essential for raising consciousness" (Griffin, 2004).

All nurses, not just resident and student nurses, benefit from education on horizontal hostility. Staff need to know what nurse-to-nurse hostility is, as well as its effects and the solutions. To start getting the message out, consider distributing a fact sheet to employees (see Figure 6.1).

6.   **Debrief, debrief, debrief!** Make this a priority every day, not just at the end of the student's experience. Although course feedback has been in place for years, augmenting this feedback with the opportunity to share personal reflections from students' and new grads' experiences will benefit everyone. Optimally, debriefing should occur at every level—with the nurse, the manager, and the instructor.

Connecting Through Vulnerability

Being vulnerable and showing emotion are considered signs of weakness in a masculine-dominated society. We receive these social messages at a very young age when we hear "man up," "girls are sissies," or "crybaby." It is ironic then that the emotions we have learned to subdue and control are exactly what we must access and express in order to bond with one another. Providing the time to reflect upon and

Figure 6.1   Nurse-to-nurse hostility fact sheet

What is nurse-to-nurse hostility?

Nurse-to-nurse hostility, also known as horizontal violence, colleague abuse, interpersonal conflict among coworkers, and workplace bullying, is a serious issue in the nursing profession that needs to be acknowledged and addressed.

Examples

1. Verbal hostility: insulting remarks, criticism, bickering, put-downs, shouting, talking behind a colleague's back, name-calling, intimidation, using a negative tone of voice, or withholding information from a colleague regarding a patient

2. Physical hostility: turning away, raising eyebrows, refusing to help, ignoring or obstructing the way of a colleague, intimidation using posture, hitting, assaulting, stabbing, or even shooting

Effects

◆ Feelings of anxiety, fear, shock, anger, guilt, vulnerability, and humiliation

◆ Loss of self-confidence

◆ Lowered self-esteem

◆ Feeling threatened

◆ Developing stress-related illness

◆ Contemplating suicide

Figure 6.1	Nurse-to-nurse hostility fact sheet (cont.)

Solutions

At an organizational level:

- ◆ Adopt a zero-tolerance policy

- ◆ Embrace a transformational leadership (with leaders who take a stand on issues, inspire, and have a positive vision)

- ◆ Develop a strong policy to deal with incidents of hostility, including a system of recordkeeping and accountability

- ◆ Develop institutional policies that are proactive, not reactive

- ◆ Develop a workable plan that gives managers the tools to act swiftly when an incident occurs

- ◆ Empower staff to speak without fear of reprisal

At an individual level:

- ◆ Gain control. Recognize that the aggressor is at fault—not you.

- ◆ Get help from your employer. Read your workplace policy on harassment or horizontal hostility to understand your options.

- ◆ Make an action plan. Seek advice from others with similar experiences, talk to your manager or counselor, and take advantage of employee assistance programs.

- ◆ Take action. Keep a detailed log of all incidents with names of witnesses. If your health is affected by these events, see your healthcare provider.

- ◆ Confront the aggressor. Make it clear that the behavior is offensive and must stop. Use the word "I" and specifically describe the behavior and how it made you feel.

- ◆ Make a formal written complain. Follow the grievance procedures provided by your organization or union.

- ◆ Take legal action. As a last resort, consider seeking expert legal advice.

Source: Jacoba Leiper, RN, MSN, lecturer at the University of North Carolina at Greensboro School of Nursing. Reprinted with permission.

express the emotions we feel in the delivery of healthcare or in school is not "soft stuff." Reflective sharing moments are powerful connectors.

One instructor who provided daily time for reflective practice said the following:

> *It was difficult at first as no one wanted to appear vulnerable or share how they felt. So I started. I started with how inadequate and frustrated I felt covering all nine of them during a particular time when I was helping with a dressing change.*

> *Demonstrating my vulnerability seemed to be the key. It was as if suddenly I had given them permission to feel. After they started trusting me and each other, they began to open up.*

> *For them, I am creating a very different scenario than what I got [as a student]: respect, dignity, and continuous learning. I encourage them to use each other as resources, which prevents them from putting others down.*

Tip	Don't miss this 20-minute talk: Watch Dr. Brené Brown on Vulnerability 2010 ted.com.

When we stop to share our vulnerability, we acknowledge our humanness. There is a great deal of strength and solidarity that comes with realizing that no one is perfect, we all make mistakes, and we all feel vulnerable or afraid at times. A formal debriefing process offers nurses an opportunity to practice being authentically present in the workplace. Instead of immediately jumping to conclusions and sulking, we can speak our truth. From our authenticity comes our power.

When speaking our truth, we must begin our sentences with the most powerful (and shortest) word of all: *I*.

> *I noticed today that you seemed bothered by my questions.*

> *I see that your jaw is set and your facial expression is stern. Did you already make up your mind?*

> *I was hoping we could explore what happened and learn for next time.*

We are no longer victims when we speak our truth because voice is a synonym for power. Responding from our authentic self is an invitation for others to do the same.

In order to grow and reach beyond our fear-based healthcare culture, leaders must focus on language and behavior (Logan, 2011). Calling out nonverbal behaviors and role modeling healthy skills in class (or simulation labs) is critical if we are to decrease horizontal hostility. These conversations are the building blocks of a new culture.

> *Yes, I was frustrated because that's the third time this week I have come onto the shift and had to run and get a new IV. I guess I should have come to you personally instead of making an offhanded comment.*

Debriefing is an excellent opportunity to elicit emotions and role model healthy responses. Without the skills to deal with confrontation and conflict, we are setting new nurses up to fail. These conversations represent the beginning of a new culture—a supportive culture where nurses feel confident and safe in expressing their feelings. There is an even greater opportunity for this culture to take hold if its roots are firmly established in nursing school.

See the problem

We are all the "culture carriers" of nursing. Our educational system is completely enmeshed in the culture of nursing and is not the problem. It can be, however, a large part of the solution if we realize that it is one of the primary areas where nursing's subordinate position is reinforced (Roberts, 1983).

Studies show that new nurses do not lack autonomy. When female nursing students were compared with female students from the schools of education, business, technology, and arts and sciences just prior to graduation, nurses scored higher on autonomy-related attitudes and behaviors (Boughn, 1992). Nor do new nurses lack an understanding of their roles (Cook et al., 2003). Thus, autonomy and a sense of identity must diminish significantly after nurses are acculturated into the hospital environment.

Students are pivotal to solving the problem of horizontal hostility because they are not yet acculturated—with new eyes, they can see what we have accepted as normal. If given the opportunity, students can recognize and articulate the practices that diminish them.

Education, therefore, needs to be designed to see through the hardly ever acknowledged beliefs, attitudes, and practices imposed on students by the dominant
group (Freshwater, 2000). Learning must emancipate students. A transformative
learning model based on critical theory, which addresses through self-reflection the
fact that many barriers to empowerment are self-imposed, can help accomplish this
goal (Freshwater, 2000). Debriefing sessions can be held in small groups and the
key points of each group shared with the class. Any exercise or intervention that
stimulates understanding through reflection is a winner. One example that you can
try for yourself, "Focusing," follows.

Create a narrative community

A useful technique for facilitating reflection is "narrative community," a concept
created by Mary Schoessler, RN, MS, EdD, for newly graduated nurses. The thinking
behind the technique is that stories are a powerful medium that give voice to
who you are. The concept stresses that new graduates need to process both their
triumphs and their failures in order to cope with their emotional responses and to
use the experiences as sources of learning and growth (Schoessler, 2005). Narrative
community seeks to create the safe space needed to discuss difficult subjects and
bring meaning and understanding to the nursing practice, as well as to increase
resiliency.

When creating a narrative community, an individual the group trusts should facilitate
the sessions. This person must listen and reflect on each participant's experience,
suggest a context for the experience, and highlight the reasons for hope. Schoessler
suggests bringing groups of 10–15 nurses together on a regular basis and setting down
some important ground rules for successful group work. Ground rules may include
listening carefully to understand and to learn, sharing stories, using "I" language,
and keeping all stories told in the group confidential.

Focusing, by Sherry McDonald

Focusing began in the 1950s when a philosophy student, Eugene Gendlin, and the distinguished psychologist Carl Rogers launched a research partnership to illuminate how humans engage in a change process. They found that the way individuals were with themselves during any kind of change process helped them move forward, resolve life situations, and be creative. Another key finding was that anyone accompanying the individual during his/her change process (such as a nurse) needed to provide a safe, nonjudgmental, empathetic presence. Gendlin's extensive research encouraged him to teach clients how to be directly in contact with their freshly felt experience, and this he called Focusing.

The three skills needed to participate in a Focusing session are:

1. Being with your body and noticing a certain kind of "bodily sensation" or what Gendlin named felt sensing. Humans have been experiencing the felt sense since the dawn of human kind (Cornell, 2005).

2. Engaging/interacting with the felt sense of the bodily sensation with unconditional acceptance, a nonjudgmental approach, compassion, empathy, and curiosity about whatever wants to express itself. You become interested in the message from your body's felt sense, even when there are no words yet (it's the body's own language). One needs to pause and wait for clarity concerning the meaningful felt experience.

3. Embracing a radical philosophy of accepting everything as it is, without attempting a fix, or without making something change, Focusing is about being with and allowing whatever wants to be known. This allowing and being present provides a safe place for change to happen on its own time and in its own way.

Empathy, compassion, and knowledgeable caring are all values in nursing (CNA, 2008), and these are embodied in the way of being with each other in a Focusing experience (Gendlin, 2007). In nursing practice and in nursing curriculum, nurses are encouraged to develop a self-reflecting process for personal and professional reasons.

New Resident Nurses

Nurse administrators and staff nurses often carry on where the faculty leave off. When new graduates hit the workplace, their idealism may be mocked and their shortcomings magnified.

—Thomas (2004)

"Recent studies of new graduate nurses have shown that although incivility levels were low, both supervisor incivility and coworker incivility were significantly related to numerous detrimental personal and organizational outcomes, such as burnout and job dissatisfaction and organizational commitment" (Laschinger et al., 2013). New graduates report that stress and job conflict are the top problems in their first year of employment (McKenna et al., 2003). Nurses who feel a lack of support and are frustrated due to intrinsic and extrinsic factors take out those feelings on new grads, and the vicious cycle of hostility continues. Anderson and Pearson have referred to this as the "incivility spiral" because exposure to hostility causes a very emotional response: anger, fear, feelings of inefficacy, loss of energy, withdrawal or disengagement, and sometimes a desire to retaliate. Mental health symptoms increase as hostility is experienced. Increasing new grads' resiliency has been shown to decrease the impact of incivility (Laschinger et al., 2013).

Thus, the first line of defense in winning the battle against horizontal hostility is nurse educators; the second line of defense is nurse administrators and staff nurses.

The strategies mentioned earlier in the chapter focused on educating new nurses, educators, and staff nurses about the realities of the floor. In addition to those interventions, new resident nurses also can benefit from the following:

1. Developing resiliency
2. Giving and receiving preceptor feedback
3. Bonding through one-on-one time
4. Practicing individual reflection time
5. Learning about and practicing responses to horizontal hostility
6. Participating in innovative programs for new graduates

Teach resiliency

Resiliency is the ability of an individual to positively adjust to adversity (Jackson et al., 2007). Nurses who are resilient can bounce back when they encounter situations that "take them down." Resilient individuals have strong beliefs, perceive life as meaningful, and are flexible in adapting to change. Since resiliency is a trait that can be developed, teaching coping strategies prepares new nurses for unexpected challenges (Laschinger et al., 2013). Asking experienced nurses to share their greatest challenge when they were new nurses, or their most recent challenge, is a way for staff nurses and preceptors to role model the coping strategies and thought processes that will allow them to thrive in their new environment. "Developing resilience-promoting environments within the health professions can be explored as a means to reduce negative and increase positive outcomes of stress" (McCann et al, 2013) and therefore decrease hostility.

Watch Three Good Things

Because we are hardwired to remember the bad stuff, Dr. Bryan Sexton developed a powerful resilience intervention. This exercise retrains our brains so that we can remember the good things. In your last two hours of wakefulness, recall 3 positive things that happened that day, and your role in making those good things happen. Fourteen days gives the maximum benefit with effects not significantly different than Prozac! (Seligman et al 2005)

To view the exercise, go to: *www.youtube.com/watch?v=hZ4aT_RVHCs.*
For more information: *www.dukepatientsafetycenter.com*

Preceptor feedback

At the end of orientation, have the new resident nurse fill out a questionnaire about his or her preceptor. This feedback, presented constructively, provides mentors with specific and detailed information. This communication is critical: It stops the "down only" flow of information and evens the playing field. It also sets the tone for reciprocity, as well as for professional and collegial relationships. Two-way communication debunks the myth that any of us are perfect. By soliciting it, managers and educators send the message that they care about the experiences of new nurses.

Informal feedback also works well. Set the expectation that after every shift the preceptor asks, "Is there anything I can do tomorrow to create a better learning experience for you?"

 Ask all preceptors to end every shift by complimenting the new-to-practice nurse.

One-on-one time

It is a well-known fact that bonding is critical and that the new grad's experience in the first two months may predict how many years she or he will stay. We have not acknowledged, however, that we have adapted to a faster work pace and have less time for bonding. Therefore, we must make an additional effort to:

- Relieve a nurse and her preceptor so that they can have lunch together and time to debrief.

- Allow every staff member to share a meal with the new resident nurse every day for the first two weeks (fosters assimilation into the group by creating belonging).

- Assign a primary coach to all new nurses for two years. A coach is different than a preceptor in that their primary goal is to establish a trusting, supportive relationship which encourages new nurses to grow: a confidant.

- Decrease a precepting nurse's usual workload tip; nurses control bed assignments. Take a group of rooms and designate them as the precepting rooms. Place the easiest patients in these rooms.

- Ask staff nurses to talk about their first day as a nurse or to share their last mistake.

Reflective practice

Encouraging new nurses to stop and reflect on their day prevents mixed emotions from building up and leading to anger. It also helps to clarify issues so that they can be addressed constructively. "Reflective practice through clinical supervision is a potential space for transformative learning to take place, to bring to awareness the conflicts between the inner and the outer dialogue, and issues of inequality and power distance that are often suppressed within the work setting" (Freshwater, 2000).

Although debriefing is usually a group process, reflection can also occur individually through journaling or peer-to-peer time. Sharing our experiences is a powerful way to connect and to make sense of our nursing culture. This introspection builds confidence and autonomy and helps us form the strong emotional bonds that are so critical to group cohesion.

Tip	Begin every class with a short story. Start with your own.

Education and cognitive rehearsal

Research shows that educating new nurses about horizontal hostility allows them "to depersonalize it, thus allowing them to ask questions and continue to learn" (Griffin, 2004). The most commonly held belief in nurses who are victims of horizontal hostility is "Something must be wrong with me." Learning is severely compromised when new nurses feel that it is not safe to ask questions in the work environment (Sternberg and Horvath, 1998). And most of all, patient safety is severely compromised when concerns, questions, and clarifications are thwarted by fear and insecurities.

In 2004, *The Journal of Continuing Education in Nursing* published an exploratory study on the effects of using cognitive skills as a shield from lateral violence. In the study, a group of 26 new nurses were taught cognitive responses that increased their interpersonal skills and enabled them to confront their offenders. After classroom instruction in which nurses practiced confrontation skills, new nurses were provided with two cards. The first card (Figure 6.2) listed the universally accepted behavioral expectations for any given group of professionals. The second card (Figure 6.3) listed appropriate verbal responses to the most common forms of lateral violence and was attached to the nurses' identification badges so that, in the event of a conflict, the nurses could reference the information immediately (Griffin, 2004).

After a year, all participants were evaluated. "There appeared to be one distinctive outcome among those confronted. **The laterally violent behavior stopped**" (Griffin, 2004). The nurses reported that they did not need to look at the cards at the time of the event because they understood the information on them and remembered what they had learned in the lecture and interactive sessions. "Knowledge of lateral violence and a behavioral action to stop it (cognitive rehearsal)" empowered nurses to successfully confront abusive nurses (Griffin, 2004).

| Figure 6.2 | Expected behaviors of those who call themselves professionals |

- Accept one's fair share of the workload.

- Respect the privacy of others.

- Be cooperative with regard to the shared physical working conditions (e.g., light, temperature, noise).

- Be willing to help when help is requested.

- Keep confidences.

- Work cooperatively, despite feelings of dislike.

- Don't denigrate to superiors (e.g., speak negatively about, have a pet name for).

- Do address coworkers by their first name, and ask for help and advice when necessary.

- Look coworkers in the eye when having a conversation.

- Don't be overly inquisitive about each others' lives.

- Do repay debts, favors, and compliments, no matter how small.

- Don't engage in conversation about a coworker with another coworker.

- Stand up for the "absent member" in a conversation when he or she is not present.

- Don't criticize publicly.

Adapted from Arglye & Henderson, 1985; Chaska, 2001. SLACK Incorporated and The Journal of Continuing Education in Nursing. Reprinted with permission.

Figure 6.3	Cueing cards attached to identification cards

SIDE 1	SIDE 2	Single card attached to ID
Nonverbal innuendo (raising of eyebrows, face-making). ◆ I sense (I see from your facial expression) that there may be something you wanted to say to me. It's okay to speak directly to me. Verbal affront (covert or overt, snide remarks, lack of openness, abrupt responses). ◆ The individuals I learn the most from are clearer in their directions and feedback. Is there some way we can structure this type of situation? Undermining activities (turning away, being unavailable). ◆ When something happens that is "different" or "contrary" to what I thought or understood, it leaves me with questions. Help me understand how this situation may have happened. Withholding information (practice or patient). ◆ It is my understanding that there was (is) more information available regarding the situation, and I believe if I had known that (more), it would (will) affect how I learn. Sabotage (deliberately setting up a negative situation). ◆ There is more to this situation than meets the eye. Could "you and I" (whatever, whoever) meet in private and explore what happened?	Infighting (bickering with peers). Nothing is more unprofessional than a contentious discussion in a nonprivate place. Always avoid. ◆ This is not the time or the place. Please stop (physically walk away or move to a neutral spot). Scapegoating (attributing all that goes wrong to one individual). Rarely is one individual, one incident, or one situation the cause for all that goes wrong. Scapegoating is an easy route to travel, but it rarely solves problems. ◆ I don't think that's the right connection. Backstabbing (complaining to others about an individual and not speaking directly to that individual). ◆ I don't feel right talking about him/her/the situation when I wasn't there or don't know the facts. Have you spoken to him/her? Failure to respect privacy. ◆ It bothers me to talk about that without his/her/their permission. ◆ I only overheard that. It shouldn't be repeated. Broken confidences. ◆ Wasn't that said in confidence? ◆ That sounds like information that should remain confidential. ◆ He/she asked me to keep that confidential.	◆ Accept one's fair share of the workload. ◆ Respect the privacy of others. ◆ Be cooperative with regard to the shared physical working conditions (e.g., light, temperature, noise). ◆ Be willing to help when requested. ◆ Keep confidences. ◆ Work cooperatively despite feelings of dislike. ◆ Don't denigrate to superiors (e.g., speak negatively about, have a pet name for). ◆ Do address coworkers by their first name, and ask for help and advice when necessary. ◆ Look coworkers in the eye when having a conversation. ◆ Don't be overly inquisitive about each others' lives. ◆ Do repay debts, favors, and compliments, no matter how small. ◆ Don't engage in conversation about a coworker with another coworker. ◆ Stand up for the "absent member" in a conversation when he/she is not present. ◆ Don't criticize publicly.

Simulating conversations creates new neural pathways. If there is a pathway for an event, created from cognitive rehearsal, simulation, or role modeling, confidence is increased. Nurses who can handle interpersonal conflict will have a cutting edge in responding to horizontal hostility.

If you know that it's going to be a difficult conversation, begin with this request: *"Will you stay in this conversation with me until we both feel alright?"*

Innovative programs

Nursing administrators all over the country are leading efforts to design programs focused on supporting new graduates.

When Moses Cone Hospital in Greensboro, North Carolina, realized that it was losing a significant number of new grads within the first two years, they developed the Graduate Advancement Program (GAP) to better assimilate new nurses into the profession. The program complements the hospital's departmental orientation and provides graduates with a yearlong mentorship with an experienced leader, who supports the student and helps him or her to build confidence and competency.

New nurses are placed in cohorts of 10 with a mentor with whom they meet once a month for a year after the initial one-week orientation. The group is a safe place for reflective practice, and the new nurses' stories strengthen the bonds between them as they share their first death or an experience with a senior nurse that was degrading. For example, the cohorts meet with physicians to discuss openly the "things that scare them." With almost no experience in dealing with physicians prior to their hospital experience, new nurses have a lot of questions, and the time with the physicians helps them decrease anxiety and build relationships.

Explore "carefronting"

The term carefronting was coined by Dr. David Augsburger more than 3 decades ago. He believed that while conflict is to be expected, too often in conflict management, situations become confrontational. Respect and concern for the individuals involved aren't considered, and participants in conflict feel personally violated.

The most important goal in carefronting is to attain and maintain effective, productive working relationships. Carefronting requires caring enough about one's self, one's goals, and others to confront conflict courageously in a self-asserting, responsible manner.

Betty Kupperschmidt, an associate professor of nursing at the University of Oklahoma Health Sciences Center, has been a pioneer in bringing the concept of carefronting to nursing practice. In her work, she describes seven basic tenets of carefronting:

1. Truthing It – use a simplified speech style, genuine
2. Owning Anger – let both your faces show
3. Inviting Change – careful confrontation
4. Giving Trust – a two-way venture
5. Ending Blame – forget finding fault
6. Getting Unstuck – the freedom to change
7. Peacemaking – getting together again

Food for Thought: Exercises

1. Interview the newest nurse on your unit to elicit his or her first perceptions of his/her workplace. Ask the nurse to rate his/her orientation and share his/her experiences.

2. Interview a faculty member. Discover his or her major challenges, frustrations, and joys.

3. Shadow a new nurse for four hours. Write down your observations, focusing primarily on nonverbal cues.

4. Write a one-page commentary on your thoughts and feelings after watching Dr. Brené Brown's video on Ted.com, "Vulnerability 2010."

Summary

Strategies designed to improve the experience of nursing students and resident nurses have one common denominator: They help form meaningful relationships. To new nurses, this connection is a vital lifeline because such relationships provide a safe place to exercise their voices. Our voice is our power. Every opportunity to express ourselves increases self-esteem.

New nurses need the freedom, confidence, and permission to verbalize concerns. Whether by using reflective practice, one-on-one time, or a retention program, they must find the support they need because it allows them to speak their truth. By doing so, they build and nourish their personal power.

Feedback from new nurses is critical, as they can best see the negative practices that our nursing culture has normalized. But nothing will change until we can openly discuss and identify the ways in which we deny empowerment. "Liberation from oppression is accomplished through a process in which education and insight into the cycle leads to connection, support, and improved self-esteem among oppressed people" (Freire, 1990).

Horizontal hostility's roots have been firmly set in an uneven power struggle. The way to break out of the cycle of oppression is to illuminate the behaviors and raise our self-esteem (Roberts, 1983). When self-esteem is low, individuals are powerless to change their situation (Randle, 2003). Thus, the very act of taking back our power raises our self-esteem.

The key to breaking out of this cycle, therefore, is empowerment. "Empowerment is a helping process whereby groups or individuals are enabled to change a situation, given skills, resources, opportunities, and authority to do so. It is a partnership which respects and values self and others" (Rodwell, 1996). This partnership between teachers and students is the new archetype we must create.

Resources

Stressed Out about Communication Skills by Kathleen Bartholomew

Creating and Sustaining Civility in Nursing Education by Cynthia Clark

"Teaching cognitive rehearsal as a shield for lateral violence: An intervention for newly licensed nurses" by Martha Griffin

"The effects of horizontal violence and bullying on new nurse retention" by Kelly Weaver

South Carolina AHEC Board Game, "Can We Talk?"(Comes with Horizontal Hostility Nursing Curriculum). *www.upstateahec.org*

Handouts, PowerPoint, Articles, Audio, and DVD: *www.kathleenbartholomew.com*

Chapter 7

Awareness and Prevention

Managers are always under the magnifying glass, with each action carefully scrutinized by subordinates ... It is crucial that managers at all levels are aware of their roles and responsibilities in upholding positive workplace environments that can increase employee satisfaction.

—*Christine Kane-Urrabazo, MSN, RN*

Learning Objectives

1. Select one way in which nurse managers can empower staff.

2. Identify two strategies to nurture a healthy culture within the organization.

In the movie, *What the Bleep Do We Know?!,* there is a scene set in the late 1400s on the coast of what is now the United States. Three tall ships have arrived at the harbor, but the villagers cannot see them because they have no frame of reference. Never in their wildest dreams would they have imagined a boat could be so huge. And so they can't see the ships. The shaman of the village stares out over the water. He has noticed that the wave pattern is different and tunes in to a strange sound. Eventually, after days and days of staring over the water, the shaman can see the ships.

And so it is with nursing leaders. Like the shaman, we must be observant and notice the small changes in our environment that reflect a larger behavior—one that is so emotionally engaging that we cannot see the profound effect it has on the work environment. As leaders, success in eliminating horizontal hostility will depend on 1) our ability to see the problem, 2) our communication network, and 3) our response.

Awareness: Ability to See the Problem

Managers are the culture carriers of the organization.

—Farrell (2005)

Researchers often use the word "insidious" to describe horizontal hostility because it has existed as an undercurrent of our profession for years. Not only is the behavior hidden, but the costs are hidden as well, as the financial impact lags behind the actual events. And when its destruction becomes obvious, it is usually too late—a high turnover results not only in a mass exodus of staff but also in a crucial break in the unit's knowledge base.

Indications of horizontal hostility

Poor employee satisfaction scores

Satisfaction surveys differ in content from facility to facility, but there are usually some similarities. The scores you should be most interested in are "intent to leave," "sense of belonging," "meaningful work," "morale of self," and "morale of others." One of the telltale signs of horizontal hostility on the unit is when staff rate "others' morale" significantly lower than their own. This is because staff who hear a lot of gossip and negativity naturally conclude that their peers' morale is much lower than theirs.

High turnover rates

This is an obvious indicator of horizontal hostility. Staff who feel that they belong will clearly want to stay—and vice versa. The key to retention is to follow up with an employee the moment you get the heads up that he or she may be leaving. Timely follow-up is crucial at this point, as the staff member's reasons for leaving may alert you to a larger problem—a problem that, if continued, could lead to more resignations.

On my unit, it was not until after a staff member left the floor for another unit that I discovered the true cause of her transfer: Two employees who ate together, covered each other's patients, and took breaks together had formed an impenetrable clique. Without the support of these nurses, her responsibilities became insurmountable.

Dueling units, dueling shifts

I was in charge of two floors. For the first six months in my new position as manager, I heard numerous complaints as staff whined they didn't want to float "there." In between the lines was the message that both floors felt that "our floor is harder than yours."

Weary of the lack of respect between shifts, I asked the charge nurses to switch shifts for a week. After only one day, the charge nurses asked to return to their normal floors, but we held firm to the original plan. The charge nurses quickly learned that the floors each had different challenges of their own, and a new respect for those challenges emerged. I never heard another complaint.

The same plan worked beautifully when shift-to-shift complaints started filtering through. "Walking in each other's shoes" was a powerful tool to help staff understand that different floors and different shifts each have their own unique set of challenges.

Presence of cliques

A clique can include anywhere from two people to an entire floor. Members of the night shift often form a particularly tight group because they depend so much on each other that group cohesiveness is strong. Years of working together result in a finely choreographed ballet as the nurses cover each other and the unit. Signs of a clique include:

- Staff who consistently refuse to work with someone or prefer to work with someone specific

- A staff member who always volunteers to float

- Exclusive meal breaks (i.e., same people, all the time, others not invited)

- Refusal to help, which results in nurses feeling like they are sinking due to a lack of teamwork

- Staff who change assignments or the schedule to work (or not work) with certain people

The presence of cliques is common in fear-based cultures. Human beings will always band together to increase their level of psychological, emotional, physical, and social safety when they perceive a dangerous situation. Managers with long tenures may be so accustomed to the cliques on their unit that they fail to act or intervene. If you have an "in group," then by its very existence, you have an "out group." There is no harm more devastating than ostracism and isolation. Last year a nurse took her own life when the group wouldn't let her in. She lived in an isolated region and it wasn't an option to find another hospital because there wasn't one for 200 miles.

If you have cliques, then you are not a team. Teams are inclusive, respectful, and communicate seamlessly with all members in an open, safe system of interactions with the common goal of providing excellent, safe patient care and supporting each other in the process. It is the role of the manager to point out the cliques, speak to the leaders of those cliques in private, and ask for their leadership and support in creating a healthy team. Hospitals, clinics, and ambulatory surgery centers are all high-reliability organizations where harm and error can be mitigated by the presence of collegial teams.

Incident reports

Be aware if these reports are always filled out by the same person or are about the same person. A nurse consistently writing up her peers may have a witch-hunt mentality. These nurses are usually very passive-aggressive—they would never directly tell another nurse about a problem. This fact is usually indicative of a much larger issue. For example, the nurse may lack the confrontation skills necessary to handle the situation, or there may be a group effort to force a particular staff member to leave. In the United Kingdom they refer to this as "mobbing." This vigilante energy can be verbal or nonverbal and often travels underground in offhanded comments. Professionals do not engage in this behavior but rather handle their concerns in private by addressing the person with whom they have an issue.

Some managers express feeling an ethical dilemma in determining if lateral violence behaviors were used to catch legitimate errors or to devalue other nurses (Hutton and Gates, 2008). But just as there is no reason to accept this behavior from an irate physician, there is no rationale for excusing hostile behaviors among staff. Managers can help uncover staff's M-O-T-I-V-E using the exercise "What's your M-O-T-I-V-E?" from AnnMarie Papa.

What's your M-O-T-I-V-E?

Think about the conversations that we have in the hallways, locker rooms, and nurses stations—the ones that involve discussing our opinions of our colleagues and their practice. Why do we have these conversations? While it is important to provide feedback and help our colleagues grow, we must consider the impact and intent of these conversations. A simple way to do that is to ask the question "What's your motive?"

Let's consider MOTIVE and ask ourselves how we can work together to make a positive impact. We know that the majority of sentinel events are related to communication. We must work to ensure that our communication is clear, concise, and constructive.

M   Mentor or malice

O   Orient or oppress

T   Team build or torment

I   Inform or intimidate

V   Vindicate or vindictive

E   Empower or embarrass

♦ Consider this. You are a nurse in the PACU. You are attempting to give report to a med-surg unit on a postop patient. That unit just had a code called and a rapid response. The patient asks when she will be going to her room. She tells you the last time she was here she waited in the ED four hours before going to her room, and the floor nurse told her that the ED always held patients there as long as they could. What do you do? Agree with the patient and bad-mouth the ED? Blame the floor for always delaying the acceptance of the PACU patient? Take the opportunity to explain that the most important thing for ED and/or PACU or any other patient handoff is patient safety and good communication. **Mentor or Malice?**

♦ Consider this: You are night charge nurse on a 40-bed medical unit. Assignments are done by the day charge nurse and are to take into consideration patient acuity, continuity of care, and nurse experience. Due to a call out, one nurse must take a five-patient assignment while other nurses have four. You notice that the newest nurse was assigned the five-patient assignment. When you ask your colleague, he tells you that the new nurse "has to learn sometime." What do you do? Do you laugh and agree? Do you privately tell him you disagree and rework assignments? Do you say nothing and allow the assignments to stay as is? Do you partner with the new nurse to help him set priorities and let him know you will both work together to keep everyone safe and well cared for? *Orient or Oppress?*

♦ Consider this: You are a very experienced critical care nurse and the emergency department nurse is calling to give you a report. The nurse is new and the report is a bit scattered. The nurse jumps from chief complaint to outcome and then back to intervention and omits the assessment. What do you do? Do you interrupt her and fire questions at her? Do you make huffing sounds on the phone? Do you listen patiently and ask your questions at the end? Do you ask if she is new and let her know she did a nice job and offer some simple suggestions for the future? Do you recognize an opportunity to improve the report and offer to work with the ED on a standardized report that works well for both the ED and critical care? Or do you get off the phone and tell all your critical care colleagues that the report you got from the ED nurse was awful— AGAIN! *Team build or Torment?*

♦ You have worked in the ICU for less than a year after struggling hard in orientation. Today, you hear the preceptor using the same pressurized tactic with someone else that she used on you. After a glowing report on a complicated patient, the new nurse forgot to mention a critical detail: the central venous line pressure. The preceptor said, "AND?" very loud, repeating herself again until everyone was looking. "AND?" Do you inform her of the effect this had on you by asking to speak to her for a moment in private? Or look the other way and allow the intimidation to continue? *Inform or Intimidate?*

♦ There are three critical care patients in the ED waiting for admission. A critical care nurse is assigned to assist. Patients are in rooms 2, 4, and 15. What do you do? Do you assign the critical care nurse to rooms 2 and 15, because this is what you do every day in the ED and you want the critical care nurse to have to see firsthand? Do you thank the nurse for coming down, discuss patients, and determine which patient load is best for all? You are pleasantly surprised that the critical care nurse appreciates being included in the assignment selection and she tells you that she can take all three patients if you can move them to closer proximity. **Vindicate or Vindictive?**

♦ A disruptive physician is loudly asking a nurse on your floor why his patient did not have the proper setup. Do you stay where you are and let it continue? Do you ride in on your white horse and save the day? Do you step forward and ask to move the conversation to a more private area? **Empower or Embarrass?**

Which nurse are you? Which nurse do you want to be? Which nurse do you want on your team? Which nurse do you want to care for your family? Clear and honest feedback is important. The way in which it is delivered is most important. Considering your motive and choosing to make the right choice will help impact the safety of our patients and the future of our profession.

Take a minute and ask yourself "What is my motive?" And make it a good one!

AnnMarie Papa, DNP, RN, CEN, NE-BC, FAEN, FAAN
Clinical Director, Emergency and Medical Nursing Hospital of the University of Pennsylvania

Absenteeism

There are many physical and psychological signs and symptoms of horizontal hostility. Frequent illness is often an indicator of a larger problem. Staff who are particularly vulnerable are those who lack support systems and usually have issues they are dealing with at home as well. Run an absentee report, and check in with staff who have more than four absences per year by arranging a one-hour meeting. Although the greatest fear is that there will be nothing to talk about after 10 minutes, scheduling a solid hour sets the space for meaningful conversation and coaching. These conversations allowed me the time to discover that:

♦ One nurse was working two jobs and sending one salary back to the Philippines to support a family with three children.

- ◆ Another nurse was not sleeping at nights. I referred her to the sleep apnea clinic. Reluctantly she followed up and was astonished that she needed an apnea machine which "changed my life."

- ◆ A mother of three small children was exhausted. She decreased her FTE to a 7 which gave her one day a week to catch up and focus on herself.

Behavior clues

Employees who are victims of or witnesses to horizontal hostility may shut down as a way of protecting themselves (Farrell, 2005). "Nurses who are silent in the workplace do not believe that their true self is being expressed, [nor do they feel] professionally independent and valued as a nurse" (DeMarco et al., 2005). Hostility decreases our sense of self-esteem. The most frequently heard comment is "I started doubting myself." The most common behavior is withdrawal.

A person who is a bully can also be a victim or a witness, as the roles interchange and shift according to circumstances. Like a play, if a powerful actor is absent, there is usually an understudy. It is the manager's responsibility to pull down the curtain on horizontal hostility.

Determining the Prevalence of Horizontal Hostility

The following are methods for evaluating staff and assessing the problem of horizontal hostility on your unit. If after assessing these areas you feel that your team is in good shape, continue to monitor the environment with the following techniques.

Use questionnaires

Questionnaires can elicit a wealth of information; you can use them to assess the cohesiveness, productivity, and psychological safety of your team. Such questionnaires do not need to be extensive, and they should always end with an open-ended question. They often help with assessment because although we might think that we have a good handle on the climate, we often do not. Because horizontal hostility is insidious, because we have an intense workload, and because this behavior has been accepted as normal for years, it often exists outside of the realm of our awareness. Simply checking in with managers or staff is empowering because it sends the message that you want to know the truth.

When questionnaires were returned, we found that nurses scored very high on feeling supported and safe. But then there were questions asking, "Can you approach a coworker about an error?" and "Can you talk to your peers about a rumor you heard about yourself?" and the answers were at the other end of the spectrum. It was very enlightening to show staff the results and ask, "What's wrong with this picture?" "Why can't you talk to your peers if you feel safe and supported?"

We found that 52% of staff had participated in a negative discussion about a co-worker in the last month ... gossip was the most prevalent overt cue and the biggest surprise was that silence, then sarcasm, were the most prevalent covert cues.

Getting to the truth about prevalence: An example

An ICU manager heard nurses making derogatory comments about other nurses every "once in a while." But when a sentinel revealed that the new nurse was "afraid of asking because they would think I was stupid," she took action. In staff meetings and informal gatherings she asked if horizontal hostility existed on the unit. And every encounter revealed the same conclusion, "No, this is a great place to work ... that stuff doesn't happen in our ICU." Then, she created a short SurveyMonkey quiz asking the same questions—but with **much** different results. Privately, staff acknowledged what they could not say publicly because group think submerges individual opinions. She then brought the results of this survey to the charge nurse meeting. After listening to the results and an in-service on hostility, the charge nurses voted to include a two-hour session in their annual education day.

Consider distributing one or both of the following questionnaires to gauge staff feelings and to assess the prevalence of horizontal hostility at your facility. You'll also find questionnaires and other resources that you can customize with the rest of the downloadable materials located at the URL listed on the copyright page of this book. Use them to gauge staff feelings and to assess the prevalence of horizontal hostility at your facility.

Figure 7.1 Sample questionnaire

1 = Agree strongly
2 = Agree
3 = Not certain
4 = Disagree
5 = Disagree strongly

	1	2	3	4	5
I am respected by my peers.					
I feel supported by my peers.	1	2	3	4	5
My work group is a safe environment in which to express my opinions.	1	2	3	4	5
If I have a problem with any member of this group, I feel good about talking to that person directly.	1	2	3	4	5
My peers respect my opinion.	1	2	3	4	5
I have good working relationships with all team members.	1	2	3	4	5
In the past month, I have not participated in any discussion about a team member who is not present.	1	2	3	4	5

What I like the most about this team is_____
_____
_____
_____

What I need more from this group is_____
_____
_____
_____

Figure 7.2	Verbal abuse survey

Please answer the following questions by circling (1) low, (2) medium, or (3) high.

1. The amount of self-esteem I normally have is: 1   2   3   4

2. The amount of assertiveness I normally demonstrate is: 1   2   3   4

3. I perceive my level of competence in nursing practice to be: 1   2   3   4

4. The amount of control I believe I have over my own nursing

    practice in my current position is: 1   2   3   4

Please circle your chosen answer.

1. In your work experience as an RN, have you ever had an experience

    in which you have been verbally abused?   Yes   No

2. How would you rate your handling of verbally abusive situations?

    Poor   Fair   Good   Very Good

3. Which of the following best describes your feelings following a verbally abusive incident? Circle all

    that apply.

    Angry   Confused   Embarrassed   Determined to problem solve

    Fearful   Harassed   Hostile   Powerless   Other

4. Did the verbal abuse occur during or immediately after a high-stress situation

    for either you or the abuser?   Yes   No

5. During one month's time, of approximately how many abusive statements

    (from all sources) are you the recipient?   0–5   6–10   11–15   16–20   more than 20

6. Have you ever taken assertiveness training classes?

Based on your experience with verbal abuse, do you believe

1. The incident had a negative effect on your morale?
    Yes   No   If yes, when? _____

2. The incident caused a decrease in your level of productivity for a period of time?
    Yes   No   If yes, when? _____

3. Such incidents led to an increase in errors?
    Yes   No   If yes, when? _____

4. The incident's effect contributed to an increased workload for your coworkers for a period of time?
    Yes   No   If yes, when? _____

5. The incident influenced your delivery of nursing care for a period of time?
    Yes   No   If yes, when? _____

Source: Helen Cox, RN, EdD, and Laura Sofield, RN, MSN. Revised and adapted with permission.

Use nominal group technique

When using the nominal group technique, a question or problem is written down on the board and team members write down their ideas/solutions. Then each person reads one idea off of his or her list, with no discussion, and the ideas are all listed for everyone to see. Team members assign points to the most important idea/solution, and the votes are tallied on a flip chart (Scholtes, 1988).

Nominal group technique is an effective tool not only with new groups but also with any staff who are stuck on a controversial issue. It facilitates input with a low level of interaction. At one facility, when managers were extremely disgruntled among themselves but would not take their issues to administration, nominal group technique was used with great success to validate concerns and develop constructive solutions.

Any intervention that encourages nurses to speak freely will not only give leaders the information they need to design interventions but will also make a statement. The questions become the expectations, and the answers will become expressions of power and enlightenment.

Clues that horizontal hostility exists can be direct or indirect. Increased complaints of poor patient care, rumors about staff leaving, negative employee satisfaction scores, and absenteeism are direct. Indirect effects include sarcasm, manipulation of assignments and schedules, disgruntled employees who are always negative, and gossip that circulates 24 hours a day. The only way to keep your finger on the pulse of hostility on your unit is to form strong relationships with key staff and maintain an open communication network.

Communication

Even among friends, starting a conversation can take courage. But conversation also gives us courage. Thinking together, deciding what actions to take, more of us become bold. As we learn from each other's experiences and interpretations, we see the issue in richer detail. We understand more of the dynamics that have created it. With this clarity, we know what actions to take and where we might have the most influence.

—Wheatley (2002)

Assessing the unit's communication network is fundamental. Hard data must trump opinions and subjective observations. Can anyone bring up any subject at staff meetings? In private? Because we cannot possibly be on the unit 24 hours a day, managers need to create a strong communication network. Creating an environment of open communication where staff feel psychologically safe is critical. Such an atmosphere invites staff to talk about difficult subjects and often allows us to get a heads up before behavior escalates.

The mob squad

It was only my third week as a new manager. As I was leaving for the day, the charge nurse tentatively approached me.

"I thought you might want to know that the night shift is really bad-mouthing you," she said. I asked her to tell me more. "Susan said you can't change the schedule because it was written into the union contract, and Deb and Megan are really angry. They said you're not touching their schedules." I thanked her for sharing the information.

I arrived at 6:30 the next day and asked to see Susan, Deb, and Megan in the charge nurse's office. To say they were surprised would be a gross understatement. To their shock, I restated the gossip that I had heard. I explained that although I had no intention of changing the schedule, there would need to be some shifting of the current schedule due to new grads—and that the old union contract no longer held.

Emphatically, I told the nurses that I would have no chance of being a successful manager without their support—as long as they "talked me down" behind my back, I was doomed. I relayed my expectation that they come to me directly with any problems or concerns and assured them that I was confident that we could solve any problem—together.

"Negative emotions will just kill a unit by demoralizing staff," I said. "They create a toxic atmosphere that no one would want to work in."

Slowly, my words diffused their anger. I realized that fear was at the root of their emotional outburst and that I needed the cohesiveness of this group.

"My plan is to have self-scheduling as much as possible, and because night shift seems like such a strong group, maybe you would be willing to take over the responsibility for your schedule. I can give you the new grad's FTE."

They agreed. When the new schedule was finished, I had to smile at the new patterns. For the next five years, the night shift nurses put out their schedule on their own.

In systems theory, this would be analogous to an "open system"—an environment where staff can speak their truth without fear of retribution. Role modeling is a critical way of educating staff and creating and maintaining an open system. If you hear a rumor and go directly to that staff member to check it out, your staff will do the same with you.

Managers can build communication skills that are characteristic of an open system by promoting the following:

♦ Charge nurse development

♦ In-services on assertiveness, confrontation skills, and conflict resolution

♦ Role modeling

♦ Building relationships with meaningful performance evaluations

Charge nurse development: Leadership skills

Getting charge nurses or key people on board allows you to communicate zero tolerance for horizontal hostility. Horizontal hostility needs secrecy, shame, and silent witnesses to continue, and all of these ingredients exist in a closed system (Namie and Namie, 2000). Changing to an open system requires staff involvement and a strong communication network that imparts a new set of values and expectations.

Charge nurse retreat

A retreat for charge nurses is an invaluable tool in building cohesiveness and leadership abilities. In effect, a charge nurse retreat is an essential time-out. Stopping to acknowledge and appreciate each other is priceless. Before the retreat, nurses on our unit felt an unrealistic pressure to be perfect and feared failure. But after nurses shared their own individual struggles with each other, they realized that "we are all in the same boat." Charge nurses stopped judging themselves and each other so harshly. The time, attention, and education devoted to the charge nurses helped improve unit cohesion dramatically.

Our most recent retreat provided an education program focused on building leadership skills. Holding staff accountable was a top priority at our facility, but charge nurses often lacked the skills to do so, so people were getting away with things.

"Go ahead," I would challenge them as we went around the table. "Give me your toughest scene; give me your worst confrontation." Then we would role-play the conflicts that were giving them such a challenge and were taking away their power. Armed with new scripts, the charge nurses went back to the unit and began holding staff accountable for their actions.

Proudly, the night charge nurse approached me the day after we returned from our skills workshop and said, "I did it! For years I have tolerated Terri's incomplete medication records, and last night I approached her with the problem it was causing and the expectation. I did it!" she said, beaming with pride. "And I thought it would take me three months to get up the courage."

Unit philosophy

At the retreat, the charge nurses all stated what they valued the most about nursing. Together they came up with a "Unit Philosophy," which they then asked all staff to sign. As manager, I explained to the staff that this unit philosophy was a product of all of the charge nurses getting together and sharing their values and beliefs, but now we needed their input.

After the philosophy was finalized, employees had only three choices: sign it, edit it and then sign it, or transfer out of the department. No one could live in the gray zone any longer. This posted document was a tangible reminder that everyone was, literally, on the same page. The following are some of the philosophy's key points:

- There will be zero tolerance for gossip and negativity on the unit.

- We respect each other. Therefore, it is the expectation that any problems will be addressed in private with the person(s) involved.

- We recognize that, in order to create a healing environment for our patients, we must create it with each other first.

- We pledge to provide the highest quality of care by demonstrating excellent clinical competence.

A unit philosophy is a powerful way to unite staff. The mission, vision, and values of the hospital are often too vague, and staff have no direct input into their conception—therefore, there is no buy-in. Creating a unit philosophy empowers staff by giving them responsibility for their own work environment. It requires that staff answer the question, "What do you value and what do you believe?"

I have your back! A sample unit philosophy

We promise to care for your loved one with the same skill and compassion that we would give to our own family members. And we acknowledge that in order to create the most optimal healing environment, and deliver high quality, safe patient care, we must care for each other. Therefore, no hostility will be tolerated on this unit. We have your back—because we have each others'.

A new belief system

Slowly, we altered the belief system of the unit. Through education and mentoring, first the charge nurses and then the staff came to believe the following:

♦ There is enough for everyone.

♦ There are things we can control and things we can't.

♦ Nobody is perfect.

♦ Every single nurse on this floor has something special to offer. If you can't see it, look harder.

♦ Everyone has his or her own story. Don't make up one before you listen to theirs.

♦ Compassion and kindness go much further than judgment and blame.

♦ You won't melt or die by confronting someone with the truth.

♦ Our greatest strength is the relationships we have with each other.

♦ Negativity poisons the work atmosphere for everyone.

♦ We are all in the same boat. Climb in.

♦ We are only as strong as our weakest link.

- ◆ It is my responsibility to take care of myself and to verbalize my concerns.
- ◆ If I have a problem with someone, I will talk to him or her in private.

Individual action plans

One of the hallmarks of our charge nurse retreats became individual action plans. With the help of the leadership cards and a peer, staff would select the three areas in which they excelled, as well as the three areas they most wanted to improve. In addition, prior to the retreat, I asked the staff nurses to fill out a form giving feedback to each charge nurse (see Figure 7.3).

Figure 7.3   Charge nurse assessment tool

Person requesting feedback _____

Circle your relationship to the person requesting feedback:

Self   Peer   Manager   I report to this person

Please rate the person on the following.

1 = poor   2 = fair   3 = good   4 = very good   5 = excellent

Quality care

1. Ensures the highest quality care and service for each person served.	1	2	3	4	5
2. Implements and monitors quality and patient standards.	1	2	3	4	5
3. Fosters a culture of non-blame for mistakes.	1	2	3	4	5
4. Points a finger at the solution instead of at people.	1	2	3	4	5
5. Applies win/win solutions to meet department and organizational goals.	1	2	3	4	5

Managing resources

6. Schedules staff in an efficient way.	1	2	3	4	5
7. Plans work fairly and efficiently (post-ops).	1	2	3	4	5
8. Is available as a resource to troubleshoot problems.	1	2	3	4	5
9. Rounds frequently with staff to assess needs.	1	2	3	4	5
10. Devises strategies to improve teamwork.	1	2	3	4	5

Figure 7.3	Charge nurse assessment tool (cont.)

11. Is a dependable resource to staff: willing to step in when there are patient care needs and able to identify them when needed.   1   2   3   4   5

Effective relationships

12. Consistently maintains a professional demeanor.   1   2   3   4   5

13. Maintains a positive attitude and fosters solutions.   1   2   3   4   5

14. Delivers feedback in a way that improves performance.   1   2   3   4   5

15. Receives feedback in a way that improves performance.   1   2   3   4   5

16. Demonstrates respectful listening.   1   2   3   4   5

17. Genuinely cares for others.   1   2   3   4   5

18. Observes and reflects on his or her own behavior.   1   2   3   4   5

Leadership

19. Consistently models service excellence commitments.   1   2   3   4   5

20. Is a patient advocate.   1   2   3   4   5

21. Actively builds relationships among staff, between departments, and with physicians.   1   2   3   4   5

22. Fosters a positive work environment.   1   2   3   4   5

23. Is easy to approach.   1   2   3   4   5

24. Acknowledges staff for a job well done.   1   2   3   4   5

25. Maintains a high sense of integrity.   1   2   3   4   5

What I appreciate the most about this charge nurse is_____

_____

_____

What I would really like to see more of is_____

_____

_____

The responses were an eye opener to all. Staff nurses had never been asked for feedback, and those in charge nurse positions had never received it from staff. Soliciting this feedback sent a strong message to staff that the charge nurses were striving to improve and needed staff input to do so. Without the opportunity to give feedback, problems may have festered, ultimately resulting in hostile behaviors.

After reviewing the feedback responses and the selected leadership cards the charge nurses had chosen, we worked on detailed individual action plans for improvement. The action plans clearly listed the area on which the charge nurses most wanted to focus, specific steps to achieve the goal, a realistic time frame, and a way to measure success. These plans were kept in a binder in my office and referenced at performance evaluations and whenever possible.

In-services on assertiveness and confrontation skills

The most effective classes are those that are attended by staff who work on the same shift. To accomplish this, I arranged for a series of crucial-conversation workshops from our Employee Learning Department and had members of every shift come in two hours early to attend the workshops. Instead of making these sessions mandatory, I explained the importance of addressing each shift's issues in the staff meetings and then asked for anyone who could not make the meeting to please let me know.

The essence of the course was that failure to speak your truth about issues—directly to the people involved—always ends up in either silence or hostility, and that neither is a healthy option. In this constructive atmosphere, staff began to share what bothered them, and then they learned the skills necessary to hold crucial conversations.

Staff reported that the workshops were extremely helpful and allowed them to verbalize repressed feelings. It was clear from the conversations in class that staff had not realized the impact that their failure to communicate had on others—and on themselves. After the first class, one of the nurses burst into my office.

"I did it!" she said, proudly. "After 15 years I finally told Lydia how her negative comments bothered me. I feel like my blood pressure just dropped by 20!"

Now she is shaking and her eyes are filled with tears. "Why did it take me 15 years to tell her that?!"

Crucial communications across four generations

Not only are we working in a four-generation nursing world, but each generation has a different set of preferences on how they prefer to hear feedback and communicate:

◆ Traditionalists (born 1925–1942) prefer face-to-face discussions and staff meetings, and are less likely to use email or texting for communication.

◆ Boomers (born 1943–1960) prefer face-to-face group meetings, and telephone calls for 2-way dialogue. Their style of communication is more open and less formal than the previous generation.

◆ Generation Xers (born 1961–1981) prefer email and texting, with direct and to-the-point communication; they dislike prolonged discussions.

◆ Millennials (born 1982–2000) prefer fragmented, short, and frequent communication via text or Twitter. They like to share their opinions electronically as well as in person.

Nurses from different generations frequently diverge in how they give or accept feedback, whether it is praise or criticism. According to Bonnie Clipper, author of *The Nurse Manager's Guide to an Intergenerational Workforce*, traditionalists like to hear feedback privately and tend to anticipate bad news. Boomers also prefer to receive criticism in private, one-on-one sessions, although praise can be given in front of peers. Both traditionalists and boomers will work hard to improve any deficiencies brought to their attention. Xers tend to take criticism more poorly and may overinterpret what is said. Millennials, although accustomed to receiving a lot of advice, also have difficulty accepting constructive criticism, but they happily accept praise in front of their peers.

And then there was Andrea. All week long (before the workshop), she ruminated about an incident that really bothered her: She had walked up to Judy, who had immediately turned away from her, leaving her feeling rejected. Andrea wondered constantly about what she could have done to offend her. It affected her mood. It affected her mental clarity. And it affected her performance. Therefore, it affected all of us. Finally, after the crucial-conversation workshop, she was able to confront Judy.

"I felt like you didn't like something I said when you turned around and walked away so quickly without saying anything. That's the second time you've done that."

"I'm glad you checked that out," Judy replied. "It wasn't anything you said or did. I was just preoccupied with wanting to get into my confused patient's room as quickly as I could after report because I was worried about him."

In another case, a charge nurse decided to stop wallowing in her usual guilt about not being able to make her staff nurse's day go better. She went directly to the staff nurse to take care of the problem.

Charge nurse: "I feel very badly about your day. Was there anything I could have done to help that I overlooked?"

Staff nurse: "No, but it means a lot to me that you asked. I get so caught up ... "

Charge nurse: "Yes, I see that, but it makes me frustrated because I end up feeling useless—helpless, even."

Staff nurse: "On second thought, maybe you could remind me to take a deep breath. That would help me slow down enough to give you some specific tasks that would lighten my load."

Unfortunately, not all nurses are holding these conversations. Instead, they are holding rejection, fear, and all the feelings that cascade forth when we fail to understand a situation. Typically, an angry nurse who sulks for the entire shift—and then projects her misery on everyone else—needs to learn healthy communication skills. Verbalizing our emotions is a lesson in empowerment. As mentioned in Section 1, many nurses have a passive-aggressive style of communication, which means that they learned early on in life to not say anything that might upset someone. It takes courage for staff who have been disempowered for years to even use the word "I," let alone to verbalize their feelings, but doing so can lead to a greater feeling of self-respect.

Hierarchy of voice

There is a hierarchy of voice that I use to encourage nurses' self-esteem. It is a "hierarchy" because each step results in greater empowerment. In performance evaluations, I share the following list and ask staff to pick 10 meaningful actions that they would like to perform to increase their self-esteem. Staff then label their choices from one to 10 (easiest to hardest). Addressing specific behaviors that are a challenge to a nurse stimulates meaningful conversations about that individual's stumbling blocks to empowerment and self-esteem.

I point out that each of the following actions incrementally build self-esteem, respect, and autonomy:

- Introduce yourself to patients with a firm handshake.
- Use "Nurse" or "RN" when introducing yourself to patients and their families.
- Educate each patient about your role in his or her plan of care every day.
- Don't apologize when calling a physician.
- Use the progress notes for communicating any areas of concern to physicians.
- Invite a new nurse or nursing assistant to eat lunch with you.
- Shake hands with and introduce yourself to all new physicians and staff.
- Expect physicians with whom you work daily to know your name. Remind them, if necessary.
- If you witness an abusive interaction, report it to the manager.
- Volunteer to represent your organization at community events.
- Use reflective practice to recognize your skills and attributes.
- Compliment a coworker every shift; recognize his or her skills and attributes.
- Always use "I" when approaching another peer with a problem.
- Speak your truth. Verbalize your feelings.
- Bring concerns that cannot be resolved to the manager's attention.
- Participate in shared governance.
- Refuse to participate in gossip.
- Don't sit by and say or do nothing while someone else is being talked about negatively. State that the issue should be brought up with the person involved, and then leave.

Hierarchy of voice (cont.)

- Identify a problem AND its solution for the unit. Then share it with everyone.
- Write an article or editorial for a newsletter.
- Make a presentation at physician rounds.
- Participate in regional nursing conferences and events.
- Speak at your nursing specialty's national conference.

Growing pains, growing skills

There is nothing as rewarding as seeing your staff grow in skill, understanding, and compassion for others. The charge nurse retreat, shared mentoring of new staff, and role modeling of confrontation skills gave charge nurses the tools they needed to create a healthy culture. Slowly, they began to see how their presence, actions, and words could make a critical difference in their work environment.

A new volunteer at the front desk was causing a lot of disruption. He was loud and talkative. He was annoying. Diane, the charge nurse, asked me if I could say something to him.

"Why don't you?" I responded.

"No way," she said stubbornly. "I just don't feel comfortable."

"Let me rephrase the question." I said. "Diane, how would you like an opportunity to grow and practice your confrontation skills?"

"I would hate it," she replied, grinning. "I hate it that you said it that way."

Together we went into my office and did some role-playing. She pretended that she was the volunteer, and I role modeled some possible scripts. Tentatively, but successfully, Diane was able to approach the volunteer with her concerns.

Fast-forward two years: Agnes arrives for the 3–11 shift. She is not just any nurse. This is Agnes the strong, Agnes the powerful. Agnes can bulldoze you with just a glance. Her words have the same effect as a typhoon. Every floor has an Agnes.

Upon hearing that she must float to another unit, Agnes voices her negativity for all to hear and storms off the floor, leaving an emotional trail of anger and guilt behind.

Diane chases her down and pulls her into the waiting area. She intends to give Agnes feedback about how those comments made everyone feel—and she does so with compassion, integrity, and grace. As a result, Agnes feels heard and understands the effect of her negative behavior.

Role modeling

Prior to each staff meeting, I meet with the charge nurses. Meetings are always an opportunity for staff or managers to bring up difficult or touchy issues—if there is an open system of communication. "A workplace is dysfunctional to the extent that unconscious forces are allowed to predominate in worker interactions, boss-worker relationships, or in leadership decisions" (Hart, 1993). I was determined not to let these unconscious forces create a toxic environment on our unit.

One month, our staff education meeting focused on the importance of positive feedback in building a healthy community. I started by going around the room and complimenting each of the charge nurses on something very specific. Then we each wrote a thank-you note to a staff member who went out of his or her way to do something that made the whole floor run more smoothly in the last week. These cards were truly appreciated by staff.

But it wasn't until the actual staff meeting that the charge nurses and staff finally realized the impact of their culture of stingy compliments.

I turned to a new resident nurse, who had just finished her three-month orientation, and asked, "Has anyone paid you a compliment in your three months here?" She was superb—confident, independent, caring, and very intelligent, so I didn't at all anticipate what happened next. With tears streaming down her face, Julie shook her head and replied, "No."

There was not a person in that room whose heart did not go out to Julie or who, after seeing her pain, did not apologize and promise to themselves to be more generous with kind words.

The key to decreasing horizontal hostility is to show its effect. **A manager's role is to bring our destructive practices from the darkness into the light.**

There are four main reasons why managers do not say what they see, or pretend they don't:

1.   If I acknowledge the problem, I'll have to fix it.
2.   This is always secondhand information, "he said-she said," so not actionable.
3.   I don't know how.
4.   Most of my staff is terrific. I only have one or two outliers.

Rationale #1

There is an inherent belief in every hierarchy that the person at the top is responsible for fixing the problems below. This was graphically illustrated to me one day as I sat in the COO's office sharing information about a critical issue when the leader responded, "Well, I don't know what's going on down there." His office was on the ground floor. The entire hospital was actually up, but the power dynamics language trumped our conversation.

> *No person, no matter how wise or powerful, can control outcomes in a complex adaptive system.*
>
> —*Curt Lynnberg*

In a hierarchy, if a manager identifies a problem, then the current corporate mind-set dictates that they are responsible for finding a solution. This is not true, however, for complex adaptive systems (CAP). A CAP is dynamic, nonlinear, and composed of many independent parts which constantly interact with each other. Organizations, especially healthcare, are now viewed as a CAP. Within this framework, the role of the manager shifts to a facilitator or guide who establishes the conditions for staff to solve problems, always saying what they see because one of the defining characteristics of a CAP is that the solutions emerge from the group.

Rationale #2

The second rationale, or thought pattern, that renders managers helpless is the "He said-she said." Information relayed is secondhand (or gossip) and therefore cannot be acted upon. In these instances (for example, when a nurse comes in complaining about another nurse), I recommend responding in one of the following ways:

1. Please bring the nurse you are talking about with you to my office.
2. How can I help coach you to solve this problem? My expectation is that both you and the person involved will report back and tell me the issue has been resolved.

This "nothing about me without me" approach sends a powerful message: that nurses are expected to hold each other accountable, to solve their own problems, and to take responsibility and ownership of the workplace. This is how managers shift the learned helplessness dynamics of any unit from parent to partner and shift power to the front line. When ratting out a peer is tolerated by managers, trust is undermined. **It is critical for every staff member to know beyond a doubt that "the manager has my back" in order to get to a place where "my peers have my back."**

Rationale #3

The third rationale for not addressing behaviors is very rarely conscious; as humans, when we don't know how to do something, we deny and ignore. The first step then is to admit that you have no idea how to get rid of that elephant that is stomping all over the place and crushing unit morale into the ground. Next, realize that it is not your problem, it is **our** problem. A manager's job is to say what he or she sees. Here are two ways you can bring the current culture to light for everyone to acknowledge:

- **Wordle it.** Wordle (*www.wordle.net*) is an especially useful tool if you work in a place where people are always complaining. Ask all staff to pick the two words that best describe their work relationships. The answers will create a Wordle cloud which you can date, print, and post (as large as possible). Repeat every two months for a year. This exercise provides a visual reflection of the work environment back to staff.

- **Print and post: What is nurse-to-nurse hostility?** Make several copies of the "What is Nurse-to-Nurse Hostility?" flyer, available with your book's downloadable material or from *www.kathleenbartholomew.com*. On the first day of every month, hand the secretary or office administrator a yellow highlighter and ask them to highlight every overt and covert behavior that they have witnessed on the unit in the last month. Then post with the date clearly marked above. Tear down and repeat the process on the first day of every month, **even if there are no behaviors highlighted**. This exercise is powerful because when behaviors are normalized, no one sees them. Identifying their behaviors as horizontal hostility is the first step to raising awareness. It is the manager's role to illuminate these negative overt and covert behaviors.

Rationale #4

The fourth rationale for not addressing disruptive behaviors is the most common: "Most of my staff are great nurses—really professional and competent. It's only one or two people, at the most."

Think of an orchestra where all of the instruments are producing a beautiful melody— all but one. Only one person is out of tune and playing the wrong notes; but the dissonance destroys the harmony of the whole orchestra. The same is true of humans in groups. And the more people who play the same note, the more the sound is amplified. It is up to managers to "name that tune."

Research in the field of organizational development has found that one bad apple literally spoils the whole bunch because when one person does not play by the social rules, or does not do their fair share of the workload, trust cannot exist (Felps et al., 2006). The impact of a single deviant cannot be minimized. Many a unit and organization have been destroyed by failing to recognize that tolerating the behavior of just one person destroys the entire team. Furthermore, when the mission and values of the institution do not match the behaviors on the floor, integrity is compromised.

Annual unit-based education

Devote two hours of annual education to competencies on communication and culture. It is not enough to just raise awareness because staff lack confrontation and conflict management skills and need new tools. Work with charge nurses to identify the top five conversations that are not happening on the unit, and use these examples to test the new skills. Begin every staff meeting with an example of a crucial conversation or communication scenario.

Figure 7.4   The D-E-S-C communication model

Feedback Formula	Rational	DESC Model (Intent/impact)	Rational
Facts First	Lead with the facts! Observable, less likely to cause defensiveness, facts are not personal. Facts are seen and heard. Verifiable by others.	Describe the situation	Describe using facts, orient the person to the issue you are discussing with them.
Story Second	Your story is your impression, your interpretation of the facts. Share what the facts meant to you. Your story usually has some emotion attached to it, the facts have caused you to "feel" something. Share your story.	Explain what this means to you	Let the person know the impact of the situation. Tell them how you "see it." This tells them why you are talking to them . . . it is having an impact on you. Share that.
Pause, Pause, Pause	Pausing allows the other person a minute to assimilate what they have just heard. It also prevents you from overwhelming the person and from speaking too fast.	Pause, pause, pause	Pausing allows the other person a minute to assimilate what they have just heard. It also prevents you from overwhelming the person and speaking too fast.
Check for Understanding	Asking, "How do you see it?" or "Do you see it differently?" invites dialogue. This step is about clarifying the situation you are giving feedback about.	State what you want instead	Discuss behavior you DO want. Be descriptive. Using the affirmative approach helps the other person know what they should do and minimizes defensiveness by not focusing on what is wrong. This step reframes the situation; "This is what I do want from you." The positive approach can make it easier for the other person to agree with you. It helps them save face.
Make a Request	Motivation is different for each person. Try to describe consequences that matter to this person. Meaningful consequences bring meaningful change.	Determine the consequences that will naturally occur if the situation continues	Describe the impact if the person does not meet the expectation you just "stated." Consequences usually have an impact on 3 levels: Individual: "What is in it for me?" What pain or pleasure is attached to this situation? Outline the benefit to them associated with complying. Social: Impact to others, to the team. What praise or pressure from others might be a consequence? Work environment: Standards, policies, rules, "carrots and sticks" associated with this situation. Progressive Corrective Action is an example of a work consequence/impact.

Educational workshops that enhanced awareness of lateral violence and improved assertive communication resulted in a better environment, reduction in turnover and vacancy rates, and reduced incidence of lateral violence.

—*Ceravolo et al. (2012)*

Do not expect staff to engage in difficult conversations if you haven't given them the tools. Nurses historically lack a confrontation skill set. The recommendations to end hostility in this book come from many perspectives and are all designed to increase esteem and redistribute power from a hierarchy to a team. But the most important of all changes must be in the way we communicate with one another.

Whenever there is a hierarchy, communication is stifled. Whenever communication is stifled, we put our patients at risk. As illustrated earlier, a culture of intimidation trumps best practice. In order to eliminate a fear-based culture, leaders must focus on language and behavior (Logan, 2008). I use the D-E-S-C communication model (in Figure 7.4) because it is easy to remember and very effective.

Build muscle memory

The audience of 40 critical care nurses had completed a two-hour seminar on nurse-to-nurse hostility followed by a four-hour session on TeamSTEPPS. To measure competency, the manager asked for volunteers to privately record the answers to four brief vignettes. Only 12 people volunteered.

In the first scene, a nurse walks into the break room and her friend asks, "Did you hear about Peggy's divorce?" How would you respond? Feedback from this group was that this scene was "Too hard ... can you start with an easier one?"

Regardless of what model you choose, unless muscle memory is built by practicing difficult conversations, then staff will not use the tool you just invested heavily in giving them. It's like offering builders the most expensive chisel in the world, and showing them a video on how to use it, but forgetting that they need wood or marble to use it. After a short time, without a place to use the tool, we discard it.

Use the feedback scenarios provided here, print out the feedback cards from *www.kathleenbartholomew.com,* or create your own. Education is not complete until we can measure or demonstrate mastery of the new skill.

Feedback scenarios for practice: An exercise

Instructions: Break into pairs. Choose one of the scenarios below to practice giving feedback as if it were a real situation. Decide who will give and who will receive the feedback first. Feedback givers: remember to be specific, say what the behavior meant to you, and pause. Feedback receivers: pretend to be someone who does not take the feedback well.

After each turn, discuss how it went: Was the feedback giver respectful? Was the feedback specific and non-evaluative? Was it clear what the behavior meant to the feedback giver? Did the feedback giver remember to pause? After the first interaction, switch roles.

Practice scenarios:

1.   You have a coworker who often comes to work 10–15 minutes late.

2.   A patient care task (e.g., oral hygiene, turning, bath) is left undone.

3.   A staff member spends too much time on the Internet.

4.   A coworker is telling you an off-color joke and you want them to stop.

5.   Your coworker repeatedly interrupts and talks over you when you are trying to make a point in a meeting.

6.   Your coworker chronically complains about _____.

Focus on the positive

Fewer than half of the nurses in Aiken's five-country study, which we first mentioned in Chapter 1, reported that management acknowledged and valued their contributions (Aiken, 2001). Managers have had a tendency to comment on "what is being done wrong, rather than what is being done right" (Thomas, 2003). "Favorable recognition was a significant predictor of job satisfaction in Blegen's meta-analysis of 48 studies involving more than 15,000 nurses" (Thomas, 2003).

Clearly, compliments and recognition increase nurses' feelings of worth and value, thereby raising their self-esteem. Encourage every nurse to draw a simple box on the bottom of their "brain" or "to do" list. This is a "compliment box." Role model and set the expectation that a shift is not complete until we have paid at least one compliment to a coworker.

Take stock of how much time you spend with staff who do an excellent job of being collegial and helpful on the unit. Share a coffee or a meal with nursing assistants, secretaries, and nurses who demonstrate professionalism. Every time you build a stronger relationship, every time you go out of your way to connect with those in different roles, you lessen the potential for horizontal hostility and strengthen the patient safety net that catches harm and error.

Performance evaluations

It is not easy to change a culture. At times, it feels like I'm swimming against a strong current. I can get pretty maudlin and discouraged trying to decrease hostility and build a healthy work environment. Sometimes, I run to my office and tap out a quick email to Oprah, which provides momentary relief. What rejuvenates me, however, are the precious conversations I have with staff—in just one meaningful interaction with a staff member, I realize again that we are *all* caught in this undertow of emotions. Every day, the pressures of our job and horizontal hostility take our profession way off course.

I once asked a peer how she was coping with the increased workload, hoping to hear some solutions I could apply myself. "I ask staff to fill out their own performance evaluations, and then I just sign them. I don't have time to meet with them," she said. I was really concerned. Had the demands of our jobs gotten to the point that we could not have just one conversation a year with our staff?

Behavioral expectations must be built into performance evaluations. If they are not, the organization inadvertently makes a statement that behaviors are not important and not integral to the safe delivery of high-quality patient care. A good nurse is someone who cultivates teamwork, brings positive energy and ideas into the group, and demonstrates the tenets of professionalism at all times.

Performance evaluations are a golden opportunity to connect with a staff member on a more meaningful and deeper level than we ever could in a conversation on the floor. If this connection is compassionate, they in turn bring that compassion and understanding to the unit. The quality of relationship that we develop and demonstrate with staff becomes the standard for the unit and decreases horizontal hostility, one nurse at a time.

A silent witness is an accomplice

Audrey is the sweetest person on our floor. She is consistently pleasant, is clinically competent, and is a team player who steps up to the role of relief charge when needed. What more could I possibly say?

A section of our performance evaluations is marked "goals." I asked Audrey what she thought of the goal I had written on her performance evaluation: "Do not stand by and say nothing while staff are gossiping. Either walk away or point out that it is gossip and then walk away." She paused and responded thoughtfully, "That would stretch me … a lot."

Aware of the fact that Audrey herself would never gossip, I asked that she take a stand. Rather than be a silent witness to the drama, I asked that she deal with negative comments made about others in an assertive manner. Then came her questions.

"How do you do that? What do you say?" she asked.

We role-played some scenes she had witnessed and discussed some scripts. The essence of the conversation was that it would take a lot of courage for her to actually say something or walk away. But the effects of "just standing by" and listening to negative comments were not benign. I focused on what emotions listening to people being criticized brought up for her. Then I asked how she would feel if she had walked away or told others how badly the negative gossip affected her. The feeling of self-respect that came with speaking her truth won by a long shot.

Summary

In summary, there are numerous ways to enhance communication and build a solid communication network on the unit. Leadership skills in charge nurses and key players are crucial and can be developed by taking the following actions:

- Holding off-site charge nurse retreats
- Encouraging a hierarchy of voice
- Creating individual action plans for charge nurses
- Creating a safe atmosphere by not listening to gossip
- Role modeling crucial conversations
- Practicing confrontation scenarios and building muscle memory
- Calling out the elephant—the behaviors that undermine a culture of safety
- Supporting the transformation from a hierarchy to a team
- Recognizing each other (i.e., using the power of a compliment)
- Increasing knowledge and awareness about others' scope of responsibility
- Instilling a new belief system, and challenging our old beliefs

Resources

The Nurse Manager's Guide to an Intergenerational Workforce by Bonnie Clipper

Chapter 8

Managerial Response

[It is] nurses themselves, who in their everyday work and interpersonal interactions, act as insidious gatekeepers to an iniquitous status quo.

—Farrell, 2001

Learning Objectives

1. Explain the manager's role in creating new cultural norms.

2. List two reasons why hostility proliferates on a unit.

A Twofold Approach

"Status quo" is an energetic equilibrium. If you take away something (hostility), you need to replace it with something else (healthy work practices). Executed exclusively, either of these actions will fail. Therefore, the most effective plan to eliminate horizontal hostility contains two critical actions. At the same time, leaders must:

- **Decrease** negativity, gossip, and a culture of blame by maintaining zero tolerance for any communication that is unhealthy, disrespectful, or spoken to people other than the person(s) directly involved

- **Increase** a climate of safety and healthy communication by role modeling and using as many opportunities as possible to teach interpersonal and confrontational skills

Nurses decide what behavior is acceptable or unacceptable by how leaders respond to it. **Our response is the only way to create new norms.** Clearly, the manager would intervene if there was an angry, emotional, derogatory outburst, but what about the covert behaviors?

> *In a healthy organization, every effort should be made to see to it that unconscious actions or motivations are brought out into the open.*
>
> —*Archibald Hart*

Some managers would think it trivial to follow up on a nurse who rolled her eyes when she found out whom she was working with that day. But it has been my experience that this eye-rolling didn't just occur on the particular day you witnessed the behavior. I will bet that it happens every day with the same nurses and that it negatively affects the work climate, taking the focus away from the patient.

To uncover covert behaviors, be vigilant. Arrange a time to meet with employees, and create a safe setting so that staff can tell you how they feel, which drives how they behave. Following up on overt and covert hostility in a timely manner is vital (even though some may argue that it is futile). Healing one relationship at a time, by taking consistent action, is the only way to communicate which behaviors are acceptable and which are unacceptable. Your consistent response is the strongest message you can possibly send, so follow up on every incident of hostility.

There is never an excuse for bad behavior

Remember that our beliefs dictate our responses. A good nurse is cooperative, collaborative, and professional in all of his or her relationships—not just clinically. Last month a manager came to me for advice. One of his peers was constantly putting him down with snide, sarcastic remarks. We discussed the situations and then developed a plan: first he would go to his director and give his director a heads up that he was going to have a conversation with his peer about her derogatory remarks:

> *I couldn't believe what the director said! Every phrase that came out of her mouth was exactly what you predicted! First, she started with, "Well, that's just the way Gerry is … she's such a good nurse … she's the smartest nurse on the unit … do you know her family history?" Then, she tried to turn it around so that it was my*

problem … that I couldn't get along with her. I had to constantly return to the core
issue which was that Gerry's disrespectful, undermining comments were personally
hurtful, destroying our team, and did not match the values of our organization.
I'm glad I was prepared or she would have just shut me down. The familiar
excuses allowed me to keep centered and calm.

Disruptive physicians

Nothing that a manager does goes unnoticed by staff—especially when they do
nothing. Addressing rude or obnoxious physician behavior is absolutely mandatory
to create a culture of trust and respect. If a manager tolerates disruptive behavior by
a physician, then staff will not believe any initiative or policy on creating a healthy
team and ending horizontal hostility. Effort to provide education on how to treat peers
respectfully is considered a joke when abuse is tolerated by management. The irony is
too obvious.

Managers must immediately go to a disruptive physician and say, *"May I speak to you*
for a moment in private?" It doesn't matter if the conversation goes horribly wrong
because if it takes place in your office, no one but you will hear it. All that matters is
that staff witness you having the courage, confidence, and conviction to draw the line.

The most common causes of a physician being upset are poor patient care or orders not
followed. Disentangle the two issues: 1) rude, disruptive behavior and 2) the clinical
issue. **There is never an excuse or rationale for treating another disrespectfully.**
Allowing one person to be exempt from this rule opens the door for more to follow
and challenges your authenticity as a leader.

When the cat's away …

In a morning meeting with the CNO of a hospital, I learned about the huge prevention
campaign that was underway due to a series of falls with injuries. Signs were posted
throughout the hospital. But after rounding on the units for only a few hours it was
extremely clear why the fall rate had increased: because vigilance had decreased.
Nurses who had a minute would pull out their personal cell phones and send a few
texts or check Facebook instead of rounding on their patients. The hospital had a
policy, but there was no one to enforce it because managers were always in meetings

or in their offices trying to work out the bugs of a new computer system. And the charge nurses did not have the interest, skills, or authority to enforce the hospital's policy.

Staff don't just suddenly get together one day, have a meeting, and decide that they are all going to use their cell phones. It just happens because one person got away with it, then another, then another … The same is true for negative behaviors. One person is having a bad day and is sarcastic and rude. If no one challenges this person's behavior and it goes unchecked, then the group has silently given its vote of approval and the behavior becomes the new norm: **"What you permit, you promote."**

Until our charge nurses developed the awareness and skills to hold staff accountable through assertive communication, changing the culture felt like an uphill battle. You have to put an infrastructure in place that supports a healthy work environment because one manager cannot successfully lead a hundred employees. One ICU manager had terrible problems with hostility and accountability on her unit—because the charge nurse position rotated shift by shift. With no requirements, job description, or training, the role of the charge nurse was a revolving door of responsibility. Until a permanent charge nurse description was created that included role modeling collegiality, efforts to change the culture had been futile. But with the right structure in place, this group blossomed into a culture of professionalism.

"Strong" personalities: Typhoon Mary

She is stocky, strong-willed opinionated, judgmental, and a damn good nurse. Yesterday, she came in early for her shift, and the call lights were going off. Very irritated, Mary turned to the staff at the main station and loudly asked, "Isn't anyone going to get those call lights?! Doesn't anyone hear them but me?!"

No one moved. Now, even more annoyed, she charged into my office ranting about the "lazy" day shift. I asked her to come back after report.

As soon as the coast was clear, the charge nurse came in my office. "I heard her," she said flatly. "But I ignored her. I just can't stand that incriminating tone of voice. I know we should've heard the lights. It's been an insane day, and everyone just sat down to chart. It's just the way she says it that turns me off."

In my meeting with Mary, it took several minutes for her to admit that no one had listened to her. Emphatically, she said that she got along with everyone—"except for the two new orientees you hired who weren't any good." Mary spoke of how she expected a certain standard of care and was not, under any circumstances, going to settle for less. Was she the only one who cared around here?

I supported her values and desire to provide the best quality care, but I disagreed with her that she got along with everyone. Although that was Mary's perception, it was far from the truth. Weary of her tirades, staff just tuned her out. Tactfully, gently, I pointed that out.

"You are such a powerful woman, Mary. Your presence has so much energy. My goal is that when you speak to people, you really stop and hear what you are saying. I want staff to know of your good intentions and respect your knowledge. I want everyone to look to you to share your great skill. How would that feel?"

Some moments you never forget. I let the feeling of being heard, respected, and acknowledged settle over and absorb into her. Like a mirror, I held up a new image—one that she liked very much. And so we began our work. You would not recognize her today.

How do you deal with loud, strong, opinionated staff? You affirm how powerful they are, harness their energy and passion, and reframe their self-images so that all can appreciate their talents and skills. Consider the analogy of a sailboat: The bigger the sail, the louder the sound it makes when there is no wind. In the past, addressing strong personalities has consisted mainly of taking the wind out of their sails, but it is far more effective to teach strong-willed staff how to *catch the wind*.

Retention of staff with strong personalities

After you set a clear vision for collegiality, those staff with strong personalities cannot survive, so they will typically go on FMLA, transfer, or leave. Injuries are common when a person no longer fits. The role of the manager here is critical in **proactively** reframing reality and offering ways to save face and advance in professionalism. Finding new, unique roles for these nurses is critical because it provides an opportunity for staff (and themselves) to be perceived differently.

Response time is critical

Last year, two children died in foster care in the state of Washington. The governor's response included a new law: Events must be reported within 24 hours and acted upon within 72 hours. I use the same guidelines for dealing with horizontal hostility.

Staff have a tendency to minimize and dismiss hostile behavior if a week or so goes by and you are still investigating. You will hear, "Oh, don't worry about it," "It's okay, really," "I'm over it," "No big deal," etc. There is a clear window of opportunity during which the hostile behavior meant something to staff. The best time to intervene is when emotions are running strong, but not hysterical. If people are extremely emotional, then rational conversation is not possible and they need time to calm down. But the general rule is the sooner the better, because events are rarely isolated incidents. Group cohesion is usually very strong in nursing and it can only be a matter of minutes before everyone distorts or sensationalizes an event in an attempt to reinforce group bonds—which is a patterned primal response.

Dealing with the cyberbully

Oh what a tangled web we weave,
When we click send, like, or receive.

Facebook boasts more than 1.12 billion users worldwide, with Americans logging in more than 10.5 billion minutes every single day. In 2007, Twitter reported 5,000 tweets a day; and in only six years, tweets jumped to more than 400 million.
Without a doubt, we have entered the digital world:

◆ Fifteen nurses received letters of warning from their State Board of Nursing after they were reported by their nurse executive for "liking" a derogatory comment that one nurse posted about a husband who was uncaring and unsupportive during childbirth. They did not heed the first warning.

◆ A nursing student was dismissed from the program after taking a picture of herself holding an unidentified placenta and proudly commenting how thrilled she was to assist at her first birth.

- A group of nurses who were friends started a conversation on Facebook which included several disparaging comments about a nurse they didn't like, as well as remarks on the safety of the organization's staffing levels.

We talk to each other on online chat rooms in casual conversations that feel so real we forget that no discussion in this virtual world is ever private. Every one of the nurses in the above situations had no idea that they were violating professional ethical guidelines by breaching confidence.

As social networking becomes more integrated into our daily lives, the boundaries between social conduct and professional misconduct are becoming increasingly difficult to navigate.

—*Rose Sherman, EdD*

While it is generally accepted that we cannot speak about our patients, even anonymously, many nurses do not realize that it is also not professional to speak about a coworker. According to the National Council for the State Board of Nursing policy on Social Media, any online comments posted about a coworker may constitute lateral violence; *even if the post is from home during non-work hours.* Communication modes for cyberbullying include: instant messaging, email, text messaging, bash boards, social networking sites, chat rooms, blogs, and even Internet gaming.

Nurses often fail to realize that deleting a comment does not erase it. Talking about coworkers is unprofessional and contrary to the standards of honesty and good morals (moral turpitude). Depending on the laws of a jurisdiction, a Board of Nursing may investigate reports of inappropriate disclosures on social media by a nurse on the grounds of:

- Unprofessional conduct
- Unethical conduct
- Moral turpitude
- Mismanagement of patient records
- Revealing a privileged communication
- Breach of confidentiality

A 2010 survey of BONs conducted by NCSBN indicated an overwhelming majority of responding BONs (33 of the 46 respondents) reported receiving complaints of nurses who have violated patient privacy by posting photos or information about patients on social networking sites. The majority (26 of the 33) of BONs reported taking disciplinary actions based on these complaints. Actions taken by the BONs included censure of the nurse, issuing a letter of concern, placing conditions on the nurse's license or suspension of the nurse's license.

— NCSBN

Guidelines for nurses victimized by cyberbullying

1. **Save all evidence.** Copy messages or use the "print screen" function. Use the "save" button on instant messages.

2. **First offense:** Ask to speak to the person in private and bring a copy of the evidence. Use the **D-E-S-C** communication model.

   - **Describe:** "I was on Facebook yesterday and my friend sent me this post because it was about me."

   - **Explain the impact:** "I was really surprised because I had no idea that you didn't like working with me, or that that was the reason you switched weekends."

   - **State what you need:** "No one is perfect. Next time could you come to me privately and let me know if you are having any issues so that we can work together to resolve them?"

   - **Conclusion:** "I am willing to learn how we can be more mutually supportive of each other for the sake of our relationship, our team, and our patients."

3. **Document** the conversation and the outcome.

4. **Second serious offense:** Report to manager (if not serious, try a mediated conversation).

5. **Third serious offense:** Report to the chief nursing officer.

Manager guidelines

1. **Verbalize that no bullying or hostility of any kind will be tolerated, including online.**

2. **Set the expectation that all staff are responsible for monitoring their virtual world.** Don't assume the parental or vigilante friend role.

3. **Educate staff on standards and policies, and provide examples.**
    - National Council of State Board of Nursing Guidelines

    - Hospital/organizational policy (including use of hospital computers, cell phones, etc.)

    - Review common myths. Use case studies from NCSBN YouTube.

4. **Be supportive of online targets and take derogatory online comments seriously.**

    Source: National Council for the State Board of Nursing: www.ncsbn.org/2930.htm

Persistence and Consistency Is Mandatory

It takes years of consistent intervening and mentoring to change any ingrained behavior. At no time can a leader "let that one go." A wise friend once told me that changing the practices or behaviors of a culture is like using the "Dead Man's Throttle" of a train: "You have to keep your hand on the throttle at all times or the train will stop." All of the above interventions, used consistently over a period of two years, began to decrease hostility and build a healthy work environment at our facility.

Along with consistency, it is critical that leaders set realistic goals. It takes a minimum of 2–3 years and strong leadership to change the culture of a unit. Many managers report that their greatest challenge however, is not endurance, but the feeling that they are losing control as tribal norms replace hierarchical traditions.

Power is not finite. There isn't a certain precious amount that we must guard with a hound-dog vigilance. The amount of power available is infinite and is a direct result of our perceptions. We don't empower staff because that would imply that somehow we give them something they don't already have. It is by relinquishing authoritarian hierarchical power that we create the conditions for autonomy, mastery, and purpose—the three main motivators for all people (Pink, 2010). Staff will automatically step into their own voice/power when managers relinquish control and eliminate the belief that some are more valuable than others.

Another way leaders can increase individual and group power is to start the conversation around the pursuit of excellence.

<table>
<tr><td>

Focus on excellence: An exercise to start the dialogue

- Ask your department/specialty to research who is the known leader in your area.
- What do the best flight nurses, critical care, med-surg, etc., do that you could emulate?
- How would you define success for your team? How do you measure teamwork?
- How could your team reach an unprecedented level of excellence and report this out in a national conference?
- What ideas do you have to raise the bar on professionalism?
- Identify an opportunity for your department to contribute to research.
- Compare and contrast best practices in the industry to your actual practices.

</td></tr>
</table>

When the pride and esteem of a few nurses soar, it raises the esteem (power) of the entire group. I encouraged and helped staff to apply to speak at their national conference. The nurses' knowledge and expertise was validated and their esteem soared when their application was accepted. They were honored and excited to be presenting, and when an opportunity for staff to speak at an all-day high school conference arose, they eagerly accepted. The nurses then resurrected their annual regional conference, which had not happened in years. Staff nurses came forward and asked if they could do it again—and put the entire conference together by themselves! A sense of group pride emerged as these events raised the esteem of the unit.

"We're a great team," the ICU nurse said confidently.

"How do you know that?" I responded.

"Because we just are … we work great together."

"How do you know that?" I responded again.

Then she was silent.

Leadership tips for collegial teams

Kathleen Bartholomew, RN, MN

- **Take a stand.** Behaviors you accept or ignore become the norms of the group.
- **Send a single message in action and words:** Patient First Every Time (The Common Goal!).
- **Focus on creating meaningful relationships... not in controlling the behavior or situation.**
- **Be consistent.** Enforce the same rules for all roles – "institutional integrity." The more exceptions you tolerate, then the more conflict you will have.
- **Always speak up.** When you see an unprofessional behavior, allowing exceptions to a standard of behavior undermines your leadership. **Say what you see.**
- **Address staff negativity directly and immediately.** Realize that just one negative employee will undermine the team by destroying trust. One bad apple DOES spoil the whole bunch.
- **Role model the culture you want to see.** Staff watches EVERYTHING you say and do, no matter how insignificant it may seem to you. Leaders bring the future into the present.
- **Ask for feedback regardless of your role:** "What do I do well?" and "What would you like to see more of?"
- **Always be honest and ethical.** Do you work with staff who you wouldn't want to care for your own family or colleague? Create a culture that doesn't tolerate poor performers.
- **Help out when needed.** This leadership action has been proven to have the greatest impact because it dismantles the hierarchy. You can't have a team if you're not on it!
- **Encourage and role model talking openly** about errors and focusing on improvements to prevent future errors. Start by sharing your own mistakes.

Remember!
To change a culture, pay close attention to LANGUAGE and BEHAVIOR. There is nothing more powerful than the language and behavior of the LEADER. When you change, the organization changes. Do something differently.

Food for Thought: Exercises

1. Select any two of the feedback scenarios or create your own scenarios. Write out how you would handle these situations using the D-E-S-C communication model.

2. Watch: NCSBN Social Media Guidelines Video on YouTube. Review your cyber activity. Is there anything you need to change or monitor? Evaluate and comment.

3. Identify a new behavioral norm that you would like to create in your environment. Demonstrate the norm. Keep a record of when you demonstrate the norm, and when you notice other people adopting that behavior.

4. Team review: What do you like the best about your work team?

5. What would you like to see more of? Identify one thing you can role model that would improve your team cohesiveness and effectiveness and write it down.

6. You are the manager of a unit and notice that a new-to-practice nurse is having trouble assimilating into the night shift clique. What do you do?

Summary

Plan of care to eliminate horizontal hostility:

1. Adopt a twofold approach:
    - Decrease hostility; adopt a zero-tolerance policy

    - Increase skills and knowledge around a healthy workplace

2. Be aware of the signs and symptoms of horizontal hostility:
    - Design a brief anonymous survey

3. Verbalize awareness of the problem to all staff—never ignore hostile behaviors.
    - Make sure behaviors are included in annual performance evaluations

4. Establish a supportive and open communication network:
    - Offer opportunities for socialization

    - Offer job shadowing of different roles or different departments or shifts

    - Use SurveyMonkey to find out if staff can openly share ideas or errors

5. Set clear expectations—hold the vision, paint the picture:
    -   "What would it feel like if every day when you walked onto the unit, you could see how glad everyone was that you were here ... appreciated for the talents, skills, and knowledge that you alone bring to our floor?"

6. Demonstrate the effect—hold crucial conversations at every opportunity. Share feedback from float nurses, preceptors, students, and new-to-practice nurses in staff meetings.

7. Education:
    -   Hold in-services on assertiveness training, confrontation skills, and conflict management

    -   Frame healthy relationships as our ethical obligation in building teams

    -   Raise awareness of the belief system that underlies the idea of a good nurse

    -   Create a new unit philosophy and have everyone sign it

    -   Encourage compliments

    -   Measure communication competency

    -   Encourage best practice and compare your unit to that standard

8. Increase the communication and conflict management skills of leaders:
    -   Mentor key staff or charge nurses

    -   Establish a strong, open communication network

9. Respond in a timely and consistent manner.

10. Make sure you have an infrastructure of formal or informal leaders that can hold staff accountable.

Resources

Changing Behavior by Georgianna Donadio (excellent book for charge nurse education)

"Strengthening Communication to Overcome Lateral Violence" by Diane J. Ceravolo, Diane G. Swartz, Kelly M. Foltz-Ramos, and Jessica Castner

"Changing Nurses' Disempowering Relationship Patterns" by Isolde Daiski

Practice feedback cards and handouts; also staff education PowerPoint and articles: *www.kathleenbartholomew.com*

Spotlight on Communication: www.comassgroup.com, 864-901-6612 (This is software to measure communication competency, building muscle memory, and virtual coaching with evaluation of competency. Also suppliers of the board game "Can We Talk" published by S.C. AHEC, including curriculum.)

Comprehensive three-hour intensive video or audio from Juice, Inc., by Kathleen Bartholomew: *www.juiceinc.com/files/documents/Healthcare_DVD_Raising_ Awareness.pdf*

1.5-hour staff training video or audio: *www.kathleenbartholomew.com*

Chapter 9

Organizational Opportunities

Social control cannot be imposed from on high;
alienation is a group trauma.

—*J.H. Clippinger,* A Crowd of One

Years ago, at a National League of Nursing meeting, Loretta Nowakowski, former director for Health Education for the Public at Georgetown University School of Nursing in Washington, D.C., proposed that disease could be best understood by looking at hurricanes. She noted that, like a serious illness, hurricanes occurred only when many factors (variables) were present within relatively narrow parameters and that an appropriate intervention could alter the severity or course of a disease or hurricane. This discovery was encouraging to Nowakowski—it meant that an intervention, made at any point, could alter the final outcome.

And so it is with horizontal hostility. Our history, gender, education, work practices, interpersonal relationships, communication skills, our organizational structure, etc., all contribute to producing horizontal hostility. The "hurricane" of horizontal hostility cannot manifest without these predisposing factors, so to intervene anywhere in this vast array can change the outcome from hostile to healthy.

The good news is that no matter what our current role—whether CNO, staff nurse, director, educator, or manager—we can implement interventions that will decrease hostility. Multiple opportunities are available at various levels.

Framework for Leading Organizational Change to Eliminate Hostility

Power is the ability to mobilize resources and get things done.

—Kanter (1979)

Enacting a twofold method (i.e., increasing a healthy environment while simultaneously decreasing hostility) is the most effective approach that managers can take to enact change at the organizational level.

To increase a healthy culture, leaders must:

- Firmly establish board and senior leadership team commitment
- Make harm visible: frame disruptive behavior as a safety issue; importance of teams:
  - Create infrastructures to support managers and staff: Include behaviors in annual reviews for all staff including physicians
- Shift the power structure from a hierarchy to a team/tribe:
  - Provide a constructive feedback system for accountability and performance
  - Provide leadership training and confrontation skills training for managers
  - Provide assertiveness training and crucial-conversation training for staff
  - Monitor the organizational climate
  - Increase social capital—build a strong informal network

To decrease hostility, leaders must:

◆ Adopt a zero-tolerance policy for all disruptive behavior:
    Same rules for all roles!

◆ Transform power from a hierarchy to a tribe/team

◆ Adopt a zero-tolerance policy for horizontal hostility

◆ Provide leadership and conflict management training for managers

◆ Educate staff about the etiology and impact of hostility

◆ Create a system for reporting and monitoring the culture

◆ Participate with other hospitals to pass state legislation

Increase a healthy culture

Garner commitment from board and senior leadership

Eliminating horizontal hostility at an organizational level begins with a team commitment from the board of directors and senior leadership. Although this may seem obvious, the concept must be restated to prevent the obvious from inadvertently blocking progress when administration attempts to hold staff accountable.

> *I tried to talk to the surgeon about his obnoxious behavior in the operating room, but he said, "I'm not employed by this hospital so you can't enforce your silly rules." How does administration expect me to look my staff in the eyes and tell them not to be rude and disrespectful when they see the same behavior tolerated by surgeons? It won't work!*

> *The V.P. took this situation to the board of directors who did nothing. At my last hospital, the board would meet with the physician and explain that if he walked through our doors, and was operating in our hospital, then he must adhere to our core values of respect … if you operate in the hospital, you* are *the hospital. What a difference!*

Commitment should stem from an awareness and understanding of the detrimental effects of hostility to morale and teamwork. Senior leaders also must realize that one of the greatest weaknesses of being at the top of the food chain is that you don't necessarily receive accurate, honest information. By its nature, a hierarchical top-down infrastructure discourages the upward flow of information. And the longer you are with any organization, the more you assume the beliefs, views, and mind-set of the dominant group in order to politically survive (which many times translates to not saying what you see). With every promotion, the eyeglasses with which we view our own cultures get thicker and thicker.

> *After hearing that I had received a job offer from another hospital, several physicians called the CEO to complain, who then called me down to his office. Since I already had a job offer, I had nothing to lose by telling the truth.*
>
> *Boldly, I said, "I hate to tell you, but you are naked. It's like the story 'The Emperor's New Clothes' ... you don't have anything on, but you think you do. At other hospitals where I interviewed, I would have half the staff and double the support, yet you keep saying that this is the best place to work. It's not."*

Reframing hostility

Hostile behaviors directly affect patient safety because cognition is impaired when humans witness rude behavior (Porath and Pearson, 2009). High-reliability teams have zero tolerance for any disruptive interactions because they understand that negativity derails communication. The prevalence of this behavior cannot be minimized: An Institute for Safe Medication Practices study of 2,000 clinicians found that 90% had experienced condescending language or voice intonation; nearly 60% had experienced strong verbal abuse and nearly half had encountered negative or threatening body language (Institute of Medicine, 2007). As stated earlier, a direct link has been proven between adverse events, mortality, error, and disruptive behavior (Rosenstein and Naylorf, 2011). Horizontal hostility is not a human resources problem, or a personnel problem, or a personality issue. It is a moral and ethical obstacle to providing safe patient care.

How safe are our hospitals? Medical mistakes (including nosocomial infections acquired in hospitals) are the third leading cause of death in America. Anyone who works in a hospital has received a call asking for a recommendation ... *"Do you know a good surgeon for my mother?"* When trust is low, people automatically access an informal network of information by calling friends who work in hospitals to keep their loved one safe. Proof that administration is aware of this inherent danger is evident in nurse managers receiving a heads up that a member of the board, or physician's wife, will be admitted to the unit—because everyone knows that once in a while bad stuff happens. **If senior leadership has not set the target at zero harm, then the expectation for patient safety in the organization will be the prevailing status quo,** which is: We are all good people trying to do the right thing, but we are not capable of perfection … But we have the best policies, procedures, and people here.

I was rounding at a hospital prior to giving a board retreat. Six patients had died unnecessarily in their system the prior year despite medication bar coding, safety huddles, etc. I asked to speak to a nurse for a few minutes off the unit, and she agreed. She was proud of her hospital and her position as a nurse for over 27 years but could not give me one example of an adverse event or error from her unit. I shared with her that the reason I was there was to help the board understand why six people had died. Slowly she reached over and touched my hand and said, "Oh honey, you got to expect some harm. After all, we're only human."

Culture is extremely subtle. A fish doesn't know it is wet.

Before buying an airline ticket, we don't search out an airline employee and ask, *"Excuse me. Do you know a good pilot?"*

Other high-reliability organizations like aviation have a different mind-set—because they didn't have a choice. When 583 people died at Tenerife in 1977, the entire airline industry was in jeopardy; when the Three Mile Island reactor melted down, the nuclear power industry realized they were all hostages of one another, because another accident would shut down the entire industry. More than 32,500 commercial planes fly above the United States every single day—so you've got to expect some harm, right?

No! From aviation to high-rise skyscrapers, nuclear power plants, and aircraft carriers, all high-reliability industries but healthcare have set their target at **zero harm**. These industries have designed reliable systems to catch error in a culture where relationships are perceived as crucial conduits of information and knowledge. Employees don't have the "right" to speak up. They have a responsibility and an ethical obligation. They understand that as humans they may fail, but by building collegial interactive teams, they can succeed (Nance, 2009). It is the leader's role to create and sustain the belief that zero harm is possible if we create a high-reliability system characterized by collegial teams.

A lack of transparency around death and injuries in healthcare has been tolerated by the general public to date because the healthcare culture has been able to keep these harmful events secret. But the push for transparency in cost, best practice, and quality will soon be followed by a demand for transparency around harm as the public shares their individual stories in our cyber world; and collective awareness spurns legislation for mandatory reporting.

What is a high-reliability organization?

By definition, an HRO is an organization that manages an inherent risk with great precision and few, if any, serious accidents or incidents ever occur. Dr. Karl Weick was able to identify a group of organizations that stood out because of consistently superior performance despite the fact that all of their environments were exceptionally demanding and contained significant elements of time compression and stress. He found that these organizations were highly reliable because the errors they experienced were caught and corrected before they progressed to a catastrophic event. Because failure of one member of the team could mean death to the entire team, they did things a certain way simply because no one was willing to risk the lives of any or all of the team members.

Common Characteristics of HROs

- High individual and organizational accountability
- Preoccupation with avoiding failure
- Broad knowledge base and high situational awareness
- Rebound quickly after an undesired event
- Consistently link cause and effect—continuous learning

("Harm Is Not an Option" *The OR Connection*, by K. Bartholomew, S. Byrum)

Keeping the truth hidden has a profound but immeasurable effect on organizational culture. A culture that is built upon secrets produces distorted, inaccurate stories which result in every employee looking out for themselves: a fear-based culture. Making harm visible raises trust. When an organization's mission, vision, and values match the everyday behaviors, the result is institutional integrity. Only when all employees feel safe will our patients ever be safe.

Zero tolerance for harm is a predicate for zero tolerance for horizontal hostility.

The critical importance of teams

Teamwork is crucial to delivering highly reliable care. Evidence suggests that improving teamwork in healthcare can lead to significant gains in patient safety, measured against efficiency of care, complication rate, and mortality (Weller et al., 2014). Recent studies suggest up to a 50% decrease in the risk-adjusted surgical mortality rate as a result of medical team training for operating room staff.

Taylor et al. (2010) surveyed operating room staff and found a perceived improvement in communication, teamwork, respect, and patient safety related to the implementation of the Surgical Safety Checkllist (SSC), a phenomenon that was also detected later through the responses of operating room staff on a hospitalwide employee opinion survey. Improved patient outcomes following implementation of surgical safety checklists has been clearly demonstrated within the Veterans Affairs (Neily et al., 2010) as well as in the Netherlands (de Vries et al., 2010) and Iran (Askarian et al., 2011).

The greatest predictor of any team's success is patterns of communication (Pentland, 2012); yet we know that nurses self-silence in order to guarantee safety in a hierarchy. Only shifting to a team or a tribe mentality can ensure that communication flows seamlessly and in a timely manner. Also, healthcare must be delivered by interdisciplinary teams if we are to survive the financial in the current system. Corporations are now selecting medical destination hospitals based on team-based criteria, for example, *"Does a team of physicians make the decision for surgery, or an individual surgeon?"* (Emerick and Bartholomew, 2013).

Furthermore, change is happening so quickly that organizations barely have time to form traditional teams in today's fast-moving, competitive, global business environment. Amy Edmonson coined the phrase "teaming" as a new way to get experts from different disciplines into temporary groups to tackle unexpected problems. And the number one behavior of teaming is **speaking up**, which is defined as communicating honestly and directly with others by asking questions, acknowledging errors, raising issues, and explaining ideas" (Edmonson, 2012).

At the core of the power shift in healthcare is transforming the current hierarchy to a team: in other words, eliminating oppression. As a complex adaptive system, solutions will emerge from teams at the point of care. However, the greatest impediment to building these teams is the belief that we already have them. Collegial interactive teams are a mutually supportive, highly engaged, continuous learning, open communication cadre of people with the patient at the center. Because psychological safety is the most essential characteristic of a team, teams are characterized by mutual respect and trust. (I like to use the word "tribe" instead of "team," because a tribe shares common values as well as norms.) If you walked into any group of humans in the world, what one question could you ask them that would tell you if they functioned as a hierarchy or as a tribe/team (Quine, 2009)?

¿poof ɹnoʎ dn ʞɔoʃ noʎ oᗡ

Hierarchy versus tribe or team

HIERARCHY	TEAM or TRIBE
Staff complain to mgr. or each other	Staff handle their own conflicts
Manager solves problems	Staff seek resolution; bring solutions
People know their place	People know their value
No feedback sought	Peer and 360-degree evaluations
Secrecy culture and blame	Harm is visible, measured, and trended
Control as key	Relationships as key
Silence	Freedom to speak up
Different rules for different roles	Uniformity and integrity

Applying Theory to Practice

Mutual respect, awareness-raising through education, development of caring nursing communications, mentorship, and non-hierarchical leadership are key to stopping disempowering discourses and practices among nurses.

—*Isolde Daiski*

As discussed earlier, the oppression theory is extremely helpful in understanding the basic dynamics of hostility and the behavioral characteristics of oppressed groups. It gives us a starting point and a framework from which to understand hostility. Now we need to view the larger picture: Hostility is not limited to staff nurses, but rather it is an "abusive and harmful activity perpetuated within organizations" (Hutchinson et al., 2006). At the heart of the matter is a diffuse and invisible force as strong as gravity: power. The question then becomes how is power given or withheld in our daily work practices?

Example: A new nurse meets with her manager and asks, "How long is my orientation?" The manager responds, "Three months." Contrast this with the manager who responds by saying, "As long as you need. Why don't you let me know when you feel ready and safe and we'll meet." Power pervades organizations in extremely subtle ways.

Infrastructure

Like new nurses, senior nurses ache for recognition in their daily work, the opportunity to tell their story, meaningful relationships with a mentor, and a set of skills that will enable them to work in a healthy environment. Yet the current infrastructure in hospitals is not set up to provide this level of support to staff. Nurses have no time for reflective practice, barely see their managers, and don't feel that their opinions matter. Their work is invisible to society, to the patient, and even to their own managers.

This situation is a petri dish for horizontal hostility. Rosabeth Kanter's theory states that social structure is critical: "Situational conditions can constrain optimal job performance and, therefore, lower organizational productivity" (Kanter, 1979). For example, a recent study of staff nurse empowerment showed that staff nurses with a chief nurse executive in a line structure felt significantly more empowered in their access to resources (Matthews et al., 2006). Clearly, adopting an infrastructure that supports senior nurses would benefit both the individual nurse and the organization in creating a healthy work environment.

With our current infrastructure, a manager has a very slim chance of being successful in the leadership role. Kanter describes power as "the ability to get things done." Most managers, however, lack time and access to resources, both of which are critical if they are ever to be perceived as effective leaders. Essentially, managers lack power. Administrative and clerical tasks such as writing schedules, fulfilling competencies, preparing evaluations, updating standards, and instituting new procedures take up such a huge amount of time that there is scant time for bonding and mentoring.

One recognized cost-reduction strategy of the 1990s restructuring was to expand a manager's scope of practice—especially in patient care areas. Span of control (i.e., the number of staff reporting to a manager, and not the number of FTEs) influences patient and staff outcomes. In 2014, hospitals are again looking at widening manager responsibilities. There is a demonstrated relationship between the number of staff reporting to a manager and patient satisfaction: The higher the number of nurses reporting, the lower the patient satisfaction rate. In an empirical study performed at a large Midwest health system, researchers also found that there was a relationship between employee engagement and span of control (Cathcart et al., 2004): As workgroup size increased, employee engagement decreased. Most importantly, **the positive effects of leadership have been shown to decrease as span of control increases** (Doran et al., 2004).

We desperately need engagement in nursing. We need involvement, buy-in, and a sense of belonging in order to establish a foundation for our work practice and any semblance of solidarity. We need leaders who can articulate and sustain a common vision, call people on their behavior, and role model new communication and confrontation skills. Without a connection between staff and their managers, the virulence and prevalence of horizontal hostility will only increase.

But research shows that "it is not humanly possible to consistently provide positive leadership to a very large number of staff while at the same time ensuring the effective and efficient operation of a large unit on a daily basis" (Doran et al., 2004). Therefore, a large span of control does not support nurses or create the structural conditions for the delivery of safe, quality care and satisfied employees. What type of infrastructure could possibly foster the level of support needed for a manager to institute the interventions discussed in Chapter 8?

Infrastructure considerations

Any infrastructure that levels the playing field, empowers nurses by giving them voice, elevates the visibility and value of nursing, and eliminates hierarchy will significantly decrease oppression, thereby decreasing horizontal hostility. **It is the struggle for a finite amount of power that provides the momentum for horizontal hostility.** But if a strong leader holds up a common vision—a vision of a workplace where everyone's unique contributions are acknowledged and valued—then an infinite amount of power becomes available. Staff united in a common goal (to create a healthy work environment) tap into a vast resource of infinite power, which in turn empowers them.

Assess nurse-patient staffing ratios

Nothing has more of an impact on the stress nurses feel than staffing levels. California mandated nurse-to-patient ratios in 2004. Yet a decade later lobbyists for unions and industry continue to debate the need for nurse-patient ratios because of mixed results. When California nurses were compared with New Jersey and Pennsylvania nurses, it was found that on average, the California nurses had one less patient each and two fewer patients on medical and surgical units. If New Jersey nurses had a similar workload it is estimated there would have been 13.9% fewer surgical deaths; a similar workload in Pennsylvania would have resulted in 10.6% fewer surgical deaths. "When nurses' workloads were in line with California-mandated ratios in all three states, nurses' burnout and job dissatisfaction were lower, and nurses reported consistently better quality of care" (Aiken, 2010).

However, another study found that while failure-to-rescue rates decreased significantly in California, hospital-acquired infections increased and respiratory failure and sepsis stayed the same (Mark et al., 2013). The lack of conclusive data on outcomes and agreement on how to define acuity have also hindered replication of staffing ratios across the country.

The pace of nursing is so volatile that acuity can (and does) change at any given moment: when the doctor tells the patient that their cancer is not in remission and their psychosocial needs rapidly escalate, or when the family of a demented patient leaves, or a nurse suddenly feels sick. It has been my experience that the charge nurses always know how many nurses are needed, but they lack power or authority. They are responsible for the outcome (safe patient care) but cannot authorize the number of nurses needed to deliver that care. This is an example of oppression—like being told that you must build a pyramid, but you can't have the minimum number of stones and mortar necessary.

Staff nurses will argue with administration (and other nurses) on the benefits of a staffing grid, but this argument is a smokescreen (veil) for the real question: Why is the charge nurse—who has the most accurate information about current acuity and nursing resources at the point of care—not allowed to request the number of appropriate nurses and evaluate as needed? Arguing about staffing ratios deflects our attention away from the fact that nurses have no authority in the matter. The lack of autonomy from staffing affects frontline nurses more than any other factor. An organization that staffs at the 25th percentile, for example, is setting the stage for horizontal hostility as well as poor outcomes and decreased patient and staff satisfaction.

Assess span of control

Employee satisfaction surveys contain a wealth of information about the climate on a unit and the supervisor's ability to engage staff. Using this information to assess leader effectiveness and span of control is crucial. Not only should low scores be noted and plans be made for improvement, but the scores for a unit must be compared year to year and directly linked to the number of staff supervised. If morale, intent to leave, and overall satisfaction scores are very low, re-survey every six months.

Shared governance

Change for the better needs to come from within the nursing profession. To develop effective strategies, bedside nurses have to be included in decision-making processes affecting them and their practice, about which they are the experts.

—*Isolde Daiski*

Shared governance is a decentralized structure in which 90% of the decisions are made at the point of service (Porter O'Grady, 2005). Moving decision-making to the bedside decreases hierarchy and therefore oppression, which alters the power infrastructure. Shared governance empowers nurses at the bedside. Nurses realize that they make a difference, that they are heard, and that they can exercise control over their work practice.

The role of empowerment in creating autonomy and job satisfaction is well known. Research shows that higher levels of workplace empowerment are positively related to perceptions of autonomy, control, and collaboration (Almost et al., 2003). Shared governance empowers nurses, and higher levels of empowerment increase job satisfaction and promote a healthy environment.

Shared governance benefits individuals as much as it benefits the organization. "Research has shown that the most cost-effective models are those models where accountability is at the point of service. In decentralized decision-making models, clinical outcomes, patient care, patient satisfaction, and patient/clinical efficacy are more advanced" (Porter O'Grady, 2005).

ANCC Magnet Recognition Program® status

Nurses in ANCC Magnet Recognition Program®–accredited (MRP) hospitals experience higher levels of empowerment and job satisfaction because they have greater access to organizational infrastructures that support them. In a study comparing MRP status and non-MRP status hospitals, greater visibility of nurse leaders, better support for autonomous decision-making, and greater access to information, resources, and opportunities were the three main elements of job satisfaction and empowerment in MRP-designated hospitals (Upenieks, 2003).

These key elements decrease horizontal hostility. Greater visibility of nursing leaders allows closer monitoring of behaviors and practices on the unit and provides opportunities to interrupt old behavior patterns. Greater autonomy in decision-making gives voice to the nurse at the bedside and leads to empowerment and an increased sense of self-esteem. Access to information, resources, and opportunities gives nurses the tools they need to do their jobs. In addition, nurses who are taught about horizontal hostility learn to depersonalize the behavior.

There are many known characteristics of MRP-status hospitals that any organization can adopt to enhance nurse leader effectiveness:

- Visible nurse executives who value nursing, and leaders who role model caring.
- An administrative team that listens and responds to staff needs, thus increasing value, worth, and self-esteem.
- Nurse executives who disseminate their power to directors/managers, thus decreasing hierarchy and power struggles.
- Empowered nurses at the bedside.
- Freedom, opportunity, and upward movement, which are the characteristics of an open system.
- Collaborative physician-nurse relationships, which level the playing field.

Manager autonomy

Education must be provided to managers so that they can lead the cultural change to eliminate hostility. According to Kanter, empowerment means having access to information, esources, and opportunities to learn and grow (Matthews et al., 2006). **Cultural change must begin with managers who themselves are convinced that they have the ability, means, and tools to change the situation.** Creating a healthy workplace culture is futile as long as managers still consider themselves victims of circumstance.

Managers have the opportunity to "paint a new picture," to articulate and hold a vision of the unit where staff are valued, acknowledged, and respected, and to approach each individual staff member who is demonstrating hostile behaviors and say, "Here, try this on. What would a healthy work environment where you were truly appreciated and valued feel like?" That vision releases a tremendous amount of power and energy.

A constructive feedback system

Providing a constructive feedback system for accountability and performance is critical because hostile behaviors flourish in a culture of secrecy (i.e., a closed system). Peer feedback, such as 360-degree assessments of managers, can be very useful. Unfortunately, these reviews also may be used to perpetuate horizontal hostility and should be carefully monitored.

Staff who feel threatened by a peer may use this opportunity for sabotage or backstabbing. Conversely, staff who carefully select who provides feedback for them (i.e., their friends/supporters) can get away with unacceptable behavior for years.

In general, however, peer feedback at all levels is illuminating. For example, the charge nurse assessment tool found in Chapter 7 proved to be an important resource for our staff, allowing them to perceive themselves through the eyes of the people they supervised. Peer evaluations equalize the playing field and establish a professional atmosphere.

Leadership and confrontation skills

"Aggression breeds aggression" in the workplace ...
and horizontal hostility becomes the cultural norm.
                                                    —Gerald Farrell

Holding staff accountable is a bedrock of quality care. What happens when leaders do not hold staff accountable? A cascade of predictable events unfolds:

- A nurse reports an unacceptable behavior to his or her manager

- No action is taken

- The nurse feels helpless ("What difference does it make?")

- The behavior continues and the feeling of helplessness is reinforced

- It happens again and the nurse doesn't report it ("It makes no difference")

- The unacceptable behavior creates negativity that spreads insidiously

- Staff who were once just witnesses of the behavior become victims of it

- The behavior is copied by others who see no consequences

- No one bothers reporting further incidents ("What difference does it make?")

Everyone in a leadership position, from charge nurses to administration, must acquire the skill set necessary to confront others. These skills, typically lacking in our educational programs, must become integral to the curriculum.

Offering education in any of these areas will help create a healthy environment:

- Assertiveness training for all staff

- Crucial conversations

- How to give and receive feedback

- Reflective practice

- Physician-nurse education and networking

- Conflict resolution and confrontation skills

Assertiveness training and crucial conversations

The void created by the failure to communicate is soon filled with poison, drivel, and misrepresentation.

—C. Northcote Parkinson (Patterson et al., 2002)

Classes designed to improve communication skills are mandatory to confront hostile behaviors. Nurses have demonstrated time and again that their communication skill set is inadequate and ineffective—they will tell everyone on the entire floor why they are angry except the person with whom they are angry. This practice is interpreted as a lack of respect and perpetuates more negative behaviors. Classes to prevent such behaviors should focus on crucial conversations, conflict management, confrontation skills, and assertiveness training.

Crucial conversations are discussions between two or more people in which the stakes are high, opinions vary, and emotions are running strong (Patterson et al., 2002)—the daily environment in most hospitals. Stakes are always high when a group must struggle for the resources they need to do their jobs (as is characteristic of an oppressed culture). Multiple opinions grow out of conflicting vested interests. When every department is struggling to stay under budget, a change in practice or a "process improvement" can result in another department having to assume increased costs. Not only does conflict ensue, but subtle task shifts often go unnoticed.

We just deliver the food trays; we don't pick them up.

I know the new food and drug interaction policy requires a pharmacist to counsel patients on the first dose, but I don't have the staff to meet that requirement.

Emotions are running strong in nursing because nurses:

- Do not have an outlet for frustration
- Do not have an opportunity to process or reflect on their experiences
- Are wounded by horizontal hostility
- Lack a support system/solidarity
- Have adapted to an increased pace of work

Because it is considered weak to be emotional in the current paradigm, unexpressed or unarticulated emotions build up. Crucial conversations are not happening, and the work environment abounds in unexpressed negative emotions. Nurses avoid conversations that "take too much energy" or handle them poorly because they are too emotionally engaged (Patterson et al., 2002). The passive-aggressive communication style characteristic of nurses also contributes to this avoidance of the issue. Nursing desperately needs a skill set that instructs staff on how to recognize a crucial conversation and how to find the "shared pool of meaning." When managers deal with conflict, the stakes are always high. Staff has a long history of feeling threatened and judged. But, as we develop our abilities to create a safe conversation zone, we role model a new skill set that encourages other nurses to do the same.

Assertiveness training and communication skills training empower staff and moves them out of the victim role. This education includes providing examples of hostility during hospital orientation, as well as offering training on how to handle these incidents. The most common pitfall of organizations is believing that because they have taught the class, people are using the skill. It is imperative that staff have opportunities to practice in order to build muscle memory and that leaders measure communication competency as they would any other vital skill.

In fact, these training methods have proven to be effective intervention tools in reducing hostile behavior in the operating room (Cook et al., 2001). Early interventions, counseling, and formal education programs to catch the behavior before it escalates (Anderson and Stamper, 2001) are highly recommended. Committed nurse leaders who use effective process and team building skills can have a positive impact on a hospital's nursing culture (Wagner, 2006).

> *Fostering an environment of lateral violence awareness, assertive communication, and collaboration can have a positive impact on organizational outcomes.*
> —*Diane Ceravolo et al. (2012)*

Recent research (Ceravolo, D. et al., 2012) supports the effectiveness of using a workplace curriculum designed to reduce lateral violence by strengthening assertive communication skills. After implmenting the curriculum, nurses who reported experiencing verbal abuse fell from 90% to 76%; and turnover and vacancy rates dropped. In addition, the proportion of nurses who believed that verbal abuse would influence their overall delivery of nursing care increased from 42% to 63%.

Another opportunity to build a culture of healthy relationships is to encourage relationships between staff and physicians. Creating social and networking opportunities enables physicians and nurses to get to know each other beyond work roles. This personal connection levels the playing field and strengthens relationships. When physician department heads and unit managers work together on hospital initiatives, staff perceive a united front and common goal.

Organizational climate

It's not about what the organization does—it's what they don't do.

—*Namie and Namie,* The Bully at Work

Culture is crucial to an organization. Like the air we breathe, it can be either toxic and poisoning or fresh and invigorating. As nurses come onto a shift, just one biting comment muttered under someone's breath can set a negative tone for the next eight hours. The toxic climate that results is not healthy for patients or staff.

Organizational climate, which is established by leaders, is a direct result of our interpersonal relationships. Thus, assessing the quality of relationships will yield a great deal of information. Do you hear frequent complaints? Are compliments given freely? What is the level of communication and camaraderie at meetings? Does each participant have equal voice, or do a few people dominate the room?

To assess the organizational climate, the mental/emotional health of staff should be measured and improvement plans put in place as needed. After assessments are conducted and the results become available, follow up with any staff who have indicated a problem. This critical step indicates to staff that they are cared about and valued.

Areas that experience high turnover and absenteeism or have many physician complaints should set off a red flag. To prevent turnover and give leaders the information they need, exit interviews should be mandatory and performed at least two levels above the employee's current level.

Social capital

Social capital describes the very fabric of our connections with each other. Over the past two generations, social capital has dramatically decreased as Americans have steadily dropped out of organized community activities (Putnam, 2000). The social capital in nursing also has decreased tremendously, especially over the last decade. The impact of increased acuity, technology, pharmacology, and patient-staff ratios, combined with a decreased length of stay, has significantly decreased social capital in the healthcare environment.

"Social capital turns out to have forceful, even quantifiable effects on many different aspects of our lives ... Networks of community engagement foster sturdy norms of reciprocity. The positive consequences of social capital have been noted to be: mutual support, cooperation, trust, and institutional effectiveness" (Putnam, 2000). Thus, it is clear that possessing a fair amount of social capital in nursing would decrease hostility and improve the work environment.

The decrease of involvement in community, in both the social and the nursing realms, has resulted in an increase in isolation and a decrease in opportunities to practice our social skills. The more productive we are, the less time we have to bond and network with each other. In our current way of doing business, if you are at a maximum point for productivity and efficiency, then social capital is minimally available. There is an inverse relationship between productivity/efficiency and social capital.

"They called me the floater," said Harry.

"What's that?" I asked.

"Well, on my breaks or during the shift, I would go to other departments and check out how they were doing. I would go to the ICU or the lab and visit. I would talk to people and, you know, check in. It was really nice. I knew everybody."

"When was the last time you did that?" I asked.

"Oh, about 15 years ago," he replied.

Social capital is a mandatory component of solidarity (Putnam, 2000). There is tremendous power available in the informal network of relationships that supports any organization. Capitalizing on this power by creating social and networking opportunities will strengthen the fabric of any organization.

[The doctor] couldn't have told you my name, despite the fact that I worked full-time on the floor for five years. Then one weekend it was slow, and he wasn't in a hurry as usual, so we started talking and found out that our kids were on the same

soccer team. Not only does he know my name now, but he looks at me like I'm a person, not "the nurse." He's so much more receptive to my suggestions for patient care.

Decrease Hostility

Zero tolerance for horizontal hostility

Obtaining honest and accurate information in an oppressive culture can be a challenge. How do you get it? By adopting a zero-tolerance rule for hostile behavior. Commitment to this policy will open the lines of communication, encourage the reporting of such events, and support the upward flow of information.

On our unit, the zero-tolerance policy for hostility came from our group of nursing assistants. After mandatory meetings designed to empower the assistants (two hours bimonthly for two years), the nursing assistants felt a strong sense of identity and solidarity. After a rather emotional week of gossip that could rival any soap opera, the nursing assistants decided that people talking behind each others' backs was completely unacceptable. They instituted a policy that if you had something to say, you needed to go to the person involved and speak to them in private. The nursing assistants wholeheartedly embraced this new policy, which was then adopted by all staff.

Staff began to realize that they could not possibly create a healing environment for patients because backstabbing and gossip made working as a team impossible. What motivated them was seeing and feeling the damage that hostility caused and realizing that they had the power to change the situation.

Why did this policy originate in the nursing assistant group rather than in staff meetings? Because the group was much smaller (12), which made it feasible to have mandatory meetings that focused on their particular issues, taught assertiveness skills, and encouraged them to develop solutions. This time together was something the other nurses clearly did not have, and this education empowered the nursing assistants.

For instance, at one of their meetings, the nursing assistants vented that they felt pulled in a million directions at once and were frustrated. When they were in the middle of bathing a patient, someone would ask them to do something else, and with a number of staff making requests, no one saw the stress of these multiple demands. So for our next class, we focused on communication skills. I taught the assistants some scripts they could use when frustrated, such as "I can be there in five minutes," or "I'm in the middle of a bath, can someone else help?"

The very first time a nursing assistant used this script, there was a loud knock on my door. An angry nurse burst into my office saying, "What bull are you teaching these assistants that they can actually say 'no'?"

When this story was shared with the charge nurses, they began to better understand the oppression within our own work group. Unit-based policies generated by staff are very effective, yet they must fall under the larger umbrella of a corporate or organizational policy in order to have Human Resources support. Also, make sure the policies are written in clear, simple language and are easy to understand. Because this is a complex subject that nurses do not wish to acknowledge, education must accompany implementation.

Education about policies must:

- Help staff understand horizontal hostility and its impact
- Teach staff how to access the zero-tolerance policy, how to report hostility, and how to find out that the issue has been addressed
- Clearly define unacceptable behaviors (give examples)
- Provide the communication skills so that staff can hold each other accountable
- Ensure that the policy has exposure on all levels

In order to support zero tolerance for hostility, behavioral standards should be included in performance evaluations. If they are not, then there is no way for management to hold staff accountable for them.

At Orange Regional Medical Center in Middletown, New York, a Standards of Performance and Behavior policy was created for all employees (see Figure 9.1). According to Nursing Director Eva Edwards, these standards highlight basic manners for employees to follow.

Prior to the policy's implementation, each employee met with his or her manager to discuss the standards and the organization's expectation of adhering to them. Those employees who refused to sign because they knew that they would not be able to live up to the standards were given guidance to help them reach the organization's expectations.

Leadership training for managers

Adopting a zero-tolerance policy for staff will mean nothing if frontline leaders do not have the leadership skills necessary to hold staff accountable. Above all, managers must be able to articulate and sustain a clear vision. They need to motivate and empower staff to change a negative nursing environment into a healthy workplace. They must be leaders.

The only way to demonstrate the impact of negative behaviors is to show the impact—the hurt and the pain—of the behavior. Leaders who have visibility and a consistent presence on the unit and who have established an open communication network can demonstrate the impact of hostility by confronting staff and holding crucial conversations. However, many nurses have become so acculturated that they fail to perceive the devastating consequences of hostile behaviors.

| Figure 9.1 | Commitment to coworkers |

"It is much easier to build a good relationship than to struggle with a bad one."

◆ We will maintain a supportive attitude with peers, creating a positive team environment by recognizing our colleagues for performance that exceeds expectations. We will hold each other accountable for our behavior and performance, recognizing that the actions of one speak for the entire team.

◆ We recognize that each of us plays a vital role in this facility's operations and treat each other accordingly.

◆ Rudeness is never tolerated.

◆ There is no blaming, finger pointing, or undermining our fellow employees or those in other departments.

◆ We are on time for our shifts, for our meetings, and when returning from breaks.

◆ We treat each other as professionals with courtesy, honesty, and respect.

◆ We welcome and nurture newcomers.

◆ We recognize that many hands make light work and offer to help each other.

◆ We show appreciation and support to staff that come to our aid from other units and departments.

◆ We do not call in sick unless we are sick.

◆ We recognize that we all have strengths and weaknesses and that it takes many diverse personalities to make a team.

◆ We respect cultural differences in one another.

◆ We praise each other in public and criticize in private.

◆ We do not gossip. We protect the privacy and feelings of our fellow employees.

◆ We profess that "There is no 'I' in 'TEAM.' "

◆ Our actions and attitudes make our fellow employees feel appreciated, included, and valued.

◆ Staff and leaders share ideas and openly communicate with each other.

◆ We respect each other's time and avoid urgent requests.

◆ We have fun and keep a sense of humor at work.

Source: Orange Regional Medical Center, Middletown, NY. Reprinted with permission.

Take a look at Figure 9.2 for an example of one organization's approach to creating a professional work environment. This organization understood that accountability must be systemwide and not limited to nursing alone. An interdisciplinary effort involved all stakeholders, began by seeking information via a survey, and continued because of support from administration which was demonstrated by revising the standard of behavior. Cultural change requires not only new behaviors, but a new language. Creation of a grass roots term ensured that this cultural change was anchored.

Figure 9.2   Case study: Creating a climate of professionalism

Professionalism journey at Medical University of South Carolina Health (MUSC)
Marilyn Schaffner, PhD, RN, NEA-BC, CGRN

As the conditions surrounding the current healthcare environment become increasingly more uncertain, healthcare systems across the nation are focusing on creating better work environments for their employees, physicians, and students. Negative behaviors in healthcare are a threat to patient safety, staff satisfaction, and staff productivity and can lead to turnover.

A survey was administered to all MUSC clinical staff, physicians, and residents in January of 2012 to quantitatively and qualitatively measure negative behavior (unprofessionalism). The survey demonstrated a high frequency of responses indicating negative behavior (unprofessionalism) is a regular issue in our work place. We started on a journey towards professionalism.

In November 2012, an interprofessional team was invited to participate in an all-day workshop. The group was divided into four major groups. The groups focused on process, communication, and accountability, addressing these questions: What would our process be for eliminating this behavior? What would be our method of communicating the change to a professional environment? How would we ensure accountability for professional behavior?

In January 2013, three task forces (Process, Communication, and Accountability) were developed involving leaders and staff throughout the organization. These groups worked hard to develop a method to transform the culture towards eliminating negative and unprofessional behaviors in our healthcare organization. Staff chose the code word "U-Turn" to be used to indicate someone is engaging in negative or unprofessional

| Figure 9.2 | Case study: Creating a climate of professionalism (cont.) |

behavior. Videos (of MUSC staff, residents, and physicians) were developed demonstrating negative and unprofessional behaviors, use of the code word, and appropriate responses. The MUSC Standards of Behavior were renamed Standards of Professional Behavior and were revised to be more descriptive of the behaviors that encompass professionalism. Response cue cards were created to promote professional responses. A Pathway to Resolution was developed to ensure accountability or staff and physicians.

The journey continues as we begin to inculcate the behaviors that ensure professionalism throughout the organization. We expect all to behave in a professional manner and hold each other accountable for the good of all staff, patients, and their families.

A system for reporting and monitoring

The very first stumbling block to reporting and monitoring is the "What difference does it make?" attitude that prevails in nursing. (If staff had seen effective actions taken in the past, we wouldn't have this problem.) **The only way staff will report the overt and covert behaviors characteristic of hostility is if they see that their reporting stops the behavior.** Mastering confrontation and conflict management skills is mandatory for managers.

Systems for reporting must be anonymous, safe, and easily available. An online reporting tool would work well. Our unit has a website with a "feedback" button that provides a secure link for staff members to send their concerns to me anonymously via email, although this option is infrequently used now that face-to-face conversations have become the norm.

Note that managers themselves can also be a problem and that a hospitalwide reporting system is optimal. Be sure to monitor red flag areas of high staff turnover, absenteeism, or high-volume patient/physician/staff complaints.

State legislation

Hospitals must seize every opportunity to advocate for legislation at the local or state levels. Addressing the impact of horizontal hostility (especially during a severe nursing shortage) at state hospital board of association meetings will increase awareness and support.

How the System Sets Up the Manager to Fail

When resources are scarce, there is always a power struggle. Thus, in an attempt to stay financially viable, many organizational decisions have been made without sufficient consideration of their impact. To respond to this problem, initiate discussions with administration that address whether the system sets up the manager to fail and what can be done to rectify the problem.

Some commonly heard replies/complaints/suggestions from managers and directors may include the following:

♦   Span of control is not being addressed.

♦   Budgets are being created with little research and without the input of nursing support staff.

♦   Bad employees are being passed around.

♦   There is no Human Resources backup.

♦   Employees are promoted and then not given the tools and resources they need to succeed.

♦   There is a highly weighted focus on productivity/efficiency—and ignorance of the benefits of social bonding and networking.

♦   Upper management has "no idea what I actually do"/role ignorance. [Note: It should be mandatory that managers follow a nurse for an entire shift once a year, that a director follow a manager through her day, etc. "I was a manager once too, you know" doesn't cut it when you held that role 20 years ago. A clear and accurate picture of the challenges our subordinates face can only result in better support.]

♦   A constructive feedback system for accountability and performance is needed.

♦   Leadership training and confrontation skills training for managers are needed.

♦   Assertiveness training and crucial-conversation training for staff is needed.

♦   Monitor the organizational climate.

♦   Increase social capital—build a strong informal network.

Food for Thought: Exercises

1. Evaluate the effectiveness of your organization's current policy for addressing disruptive behavior.

2. Evaluate the span of control for managers in your organization.

3. Ask a member of the board of directors to follow you for a four-hour shift. Compile a summary of your observations, and note their observations as well.

4. If the behaviors you see on your unit do not match the vision and values of your hospital, then make an appointment with the chief medical officer or chief nursing officer of your institution to identify solutions to the discrepancy.

Summary

Organizational strategies

1. Establish visible senior leadership team commitment
    - Communicate the vision of a healthy work environment

2. Assess and address infrastructure needs
    - Use the wealth of information available in employee satisfaction surveys
    - Pursue a shared governance model/MRP status
    - Reexamine span of control

3. Institute policies
    - Adopt a zero-tolerance policy for horizontal hostility
    - Include behavioral standards in performance evaluations
    - Require mandatory exit interviews with managers/leaders who are two levels above the employee's level

4. Provide education
    - Create opportunities for reflective practice
    - Provide classes on assertiveness training and crucial conversations
    - Provide opportunities for physician-nurse education and networking
    - Provide conflict management and confrontation skills classes for managers/leaders, as well as intense leadership training

5. Assess the cohesiveness and psychological safety of work groups
    –   Use nominal group technique or anonymous surveys to elicit information

    –   Create an anonymous reporting system, and monitor red-flag areas closely

6. Provide opportunities to increase social support network/bonding
    –   Make sure meetings include time to bond

    –   Make sure meetings are not simply a place to disseminate information

    –   Give managers and directors the opportunity to speak about their individual challenges and solutions

7. Participate with other hospitals to pass zero-tolerance legislation to protect nurses from hostility from peers, patients, and visitors

Resources

Changing Nurses' Disempowering Relationship Patterns by Isolde Daiski

Crucial Conversation: Tools for Talking When Stakes Are High by Kerry Patterson

Fierce Conversations: Achieving Success at Work & in Life, One Conversation at a Time by Susan Scott

Juice: The Power of Conversation: The Secret to Releasing Your People's Brilliance and Expanding Your Leadership Influence by Brady G. Wilson

Chapter 10

Individual Response

We're creating the future every day, by what we choose to do.
If we want a different future, we have to take responsibility for
what we are doing in the present.
—Wheatley (2002)

Learning Objectives

1. Identify two practices or behaviors characteristic of an open system.

2. Explain how you will be a leader in the cultural transformation of nursing.

Starting With Ourselves

After giving a speech at a small community hospital, I invited the audience to contact me with their stories of horizontal hostility. Immediately after I finished, five nurses came up to the front of the room to share their own experiences. Four of them were brand-new nurses. Concerned, I looked for the right moment to share this important information with the director.

"Did you notice the new grads coming up to the front of the room offering examples of horizontal hostility? They seemed pretty anxious to tell their stories."

"Did you see all the happy faces leaving the room?" she said, completely ignoring my remark.

"And yesterday was the same way," she continued. "It's so good to see the smiles on the nurses' faces as they leave the retreat."

A few weeks later, I had lunch with a colleague of the director and told her what had happened.

"She's just overworked," the colleague replied. "There's a new computer project. She probably works 70 hours a week now. She just couldn't hear you," she said plainly.

And then she added, "She can't hear me either."

Before we begin illuminating the behavior of others, we must first illuminate our own. Regardless of our position, from educator to CNO to staff nurse, taking a minute to assess the role we play in ending or perpetuating horizontal hostility in the workplace is critical. This is especially difficult in light of recent research, which has discovered that as humans we consistently rate ourselves higher than our peers would rate us, seeking out evidence that confirms what we want to believe. The more educated we are, for example, the less willing we are to correct our false opinion, because we are so confident that we are right about everything (Haidt, 2012). Self-evaluation takes leadership and courage.

Unfortunately, apathy, denial, indifference, or being totally overwhelmed and unavailable are commonly reported leadership reactions to horizontal hostility. Research shows that staff nurses do not feel that telling a manager about hostility is an effective solution. After experiencing verbal abuse, 78% talk to a friend and 32% talk to a manager—but 10% of that 32% say that talking to a manager is of no help (Farrell, 2005).

Therefore, the insidious nature of horizontal hostility is the greatest problem. Starting with ourselves, we need to create a new norm. To bring hostility to light, we must show its effect. By doing so, the healing process can begin and genuine relationships can begin to take root. Every one of the thousands of stories I have heard in the last decade have not only been heartbreaking, but they have put our patients in clear and imminent danger.

I'm an ICU nurse and my patient was crashing. I ran out of the room and asked for help from the first nurse I saw but she responded, "Sorry, going on smoke break." Only two of our nurses are like this, and when they are on the schedule with me I literally get sick to my stomach with apprehension knowing I am on my own … the manager is her best friend … please don't say anything, as this hospital is so much better than the last.

I feel so bad. I put my baby in danger because of my own insecurities. Last time I had called the respiratory therapist he said, "What are you, a two-year nurse? You could have handled this by yourself." So the next time, rather than call for help, I allowed my baby's breathing to be severely compromised—I put my baby in danger because I didn't want to be put down again.

As nurses tell me these stories, I watch their body language. They clutch their stomachs and their eyes shoot down to the floor, which is how all humans express shame. Anger, fear, blame, pride … these emotions were designed as a mechanism for survival of our species. As neurobiologist Antonio Demasio says: "Emotions are themselves a kind of intelligence. They signal what is important, desirable, and dangerous, and act as motivators and governors of cognitive and physical activity."

Emotions govern our behavior and are biologically based. Ignoring them does not make them go away. If we could only validate these powerful emotions and listen to the messages they are sending, we could truly evolve—as a profession and a species. Feelings are not "weak stuff." And as we take care of our individual relationships with the same compassion that we demonstrate to our patients, a strength and power as never seen before will emerge. As these meaningful relationships grow, not only will horizontal hostility decrease, but the solidarity we so desperately need to bring healing to a sick world will increase.

Ideas are crystallized by emotion.

—*Jonathan Haidt*

Courageous Leadership

Every nurse must lead this cultural change. It always takes a tremendous amount of moral courage to go against the norms. After managing my unit for six years, I returned as a per diem staff nurse for the next four years. I love bedside nursing and was curious: Were the changes I had made as a leader on the floor truly sustained cultural change? How could I continue to lead from a frontline staff position?

I read once that when a profession loses its uniform, it loses its identity. And so every day I wore a white lab coat with my name and degrees embroidered in red. I only wore all white, or solid navy blue with the lab coat. Every single shift at least one of my patients would make a positive comment. The most frequent one was, "Oh, I have a real nurse today." I could see the relief on their faces as soon as I walked in the room as my outfit reinforced my feelings of professionalism and my patient's trust.

But even my tenure as manager did not make the crucial conversations I needed to have with physicians and staff at times any easier. There were numerous situations where I literally had to force myself to speak up when an assignment was unfair or a physician was belittling. Bucking the status quo is never easy. I felt proud to be a member of such a great team and accepted—albeit still teased about my uniform. Together we had successfully created a new set of norms that supported each other and our patients.

Through these team efforts, we created a work environment with significantly reduced oppression. Were we able to eradicate it completely? Unfortunately, not, because hospitals themselves are oppressed in the current business model as they struggle to shift from volume- to value-based care. Nurses still encountered situations related to staffing and resources where they were overwhelmed with a heavy patient load. But we knew too much to take our frustrations out on each other.

As in many institutions, nurses find themselves trapped in an archaic business model where finances and control trump autonomous quality care. They are trusted to take care of the patient but not trusted enough to decide the level of staffing needed to deliver that care. Just as staff nurses have internalized overt and covert behaviors as normal, hospital leaders have internalized practices that unconsciously perpetuate oppression. The chances are slim, however, that management is actually aware of these behaviors because, like all humans, we have assimilated into our roles:

> I was exasperated. In tears, I turned the corner and accidentally bumped into the vice president of human resources. "What's the matter?" she asked. I didn't know where to start. "We've had a 35% turnover in our manager group in less than a year. How high does that number have to be before you notice ... before somebody cares? 50%? 100%?"

I told my director about the backstabbing and gossip. She was useless—turned it right back on me. Her only response was, "Now why do you think someone would be so mean to you?"

Due to the pressures outlined in Section 1—including the power struggle that results from a scarcity of resources—nursing administration functions as a closed system, and closed systems are by their very nature dysfunctional.

Experienced nurses are very familiar with the story of the bucket of crabs. A man was walking by and saw a crab starting to crawl up and out of the bucket. Quickly, he told the kids, "You better put a lid on those crabs or they'll get out." But the kids responded, "Mister, everyone knows you don't need a lid on a bucket of crabs because every time one tries to escape, the other crabs pull it back down."

Like a bucket of crabs, any group of oppressed people will use degrading and dehumanizing overt and covert tactics to ensure that all members of the group are oppressed. There seems to be an unwritten rule that says, "If I have no power and am stuck in this mess, then everyone else should be too."

The chief nursing officer listened intently to my presentation on "Healing Nurse-to-Nurse Hostility." Afterward, she asked the audience if anyone had any questions; but the room was silent. No one wanted to crawl out of this bucket—or even admit there was a bucket!

"I have a question," she said finally, turning somberly to address me. "I looked the other way when these behaviors occurred in the past. How do I reverse course and start addressing negative acts now and still have any credibility? People might perceive me as a hypocrite."

"You speak your truth," I replied. "You say, 'I tolerated these behaviors in the past because I had no idea how damaging they were to our patients, and to each other. In the future, I will not tolerate any overt or covert behaviors—and if you ever see them in me, please let me know.'"

This is how one nursing leader kicked over the bucket of crabs. She was transparent, genuine, and had the courage to share her own personal story. Leaders like this nurse set the conditions for change to emerge from the grass roots by addressing behaviors that threaten trust. Trust fosters a positive learning environment, which can only take place when people feel safe, mentally in tune with their leader, and truly engaged—

as demonstrated by studies using magnetic imaging. It is the way we are wired as humans.

There Is Nothing More Powerful Than Your Own Story

I am Marie. That is my middle name. When I first wrote this book in deference to my peers, I portrayed my experiences anonymously out of respect. Now that almost a decade has passed, I can share with you that the most difficult challenge in writing this book was that this process forced me to look at my own pain. And the greatest relief came from the realization that there wasn't something wrong or inadequate with me that caused the group to push me away and reject me. They didn't know what they were doing. Culture and power are subtle yet powerful drivers of human behavior.

Understanding horizontal hostility allows us to not only have compassion for ourselves, but for all the players stuck in the same drama, regardless of their role. Nurses blame each other and their managers, who blame their directors, who blame the CNO, who can't even find who to blame for the scarcity of resources and dysfunctional system. "They" are all hiding in the shadows of the corporate culture. To paraphrase Pogo (in the comic strip), "We have met the enemy, and 'they' is us."

> To look at the shadow is to intentionally address what is hidden, repressed, or denied. Shadow work is essential for self-discovery. What is hidden in the unconscious keeps the nurse from accounting for behavior like aggression and compulsivity which shows up as sabotage, manipulation, and workaholism …
> it is easier to project denied aspects onto others than to admit our own.
>
> — *Elizabeth Robinson*, The Soul of the Nurse

Leading Open Systems

> The real tragedy is that when nurses suffer, patients suffer. And when decisions about the future of health care are made without the knowledge and wisdom of nurses, quality of care will deteriorate. If we do not stop the infighting, rally around this incredible profession, and form a powerful governing body representing a single workforce of three million strong, we will have failed to rescue ourselves.
>
> —*Bartholomew (2010)*

One common observation from outsiders is the above and beyond amount of effort that nursing administrators typically pour into their work. Many nurse leaders go far beyond the call of duty—often to the point of exhaustion. This dedication is yet another cultural meme of nursing and is actually detrimental. If we are constantly plugging the holes in the dam, no one will ever notice that it is broken and leaking (for example, not charging for overtime). We don't need to work any harder; we need to challenge the system structure itself. Overworking is a characteristic of a closed system. Other characteristics of a closed system include:

♦ Little professional or social contact with similar groups

♦ Treating outsider and individual opinions with suspicion

♦ Worker dysfunction, passed on from generation to generation

♦ An expectation that one must surrender one's personal and family life out of loyalty

♦ Increased dependence on the job for social support (Hart, 1993)

♦ Fear of saying what one really thinks

♦ Little to no social interaction

♦ All conversations at breaks or meal times dominated by work issues

Creating an open system would benefit administrators, nurse managers, educators, and staff alike, but it requires that we redefine our beliefs and boundaries. Characteristics of an open system include:

♦ Mandatory "time-outs" at meetings for open forum, networking, or out-of-the-box thinking

♦ The sharing of struggles (e.g., brainstorming for solutions together, taking the time to share problems, and taking pride in the solutions)

♦ Communication that flows freely; proficiency at addressing conflict and confrontations

♦ Reasonable work hours

♦ Time and support to participate in professional groups

♦ Reasonable scope of practice

♦ The freedom, ability, and safety to say no and have it be heard

- Mutual respect and admiration (i.e., zero cliques and zero gossip)

- Leaders who report being energized from being in one another's presence

Leadership Framework

We tell ourselves stories in order to live. Of all our stories, it is the scientific ones that most define us. Those stories create our perception of the universe and how it operates; and from this we shape all our societal structures; our relationships with each other and our environment, methods of doing business, education …
defining our borders and our planet.

—*Joan Didion,* The Field

Nothing is more critical than the conceptual framework we use to frame our reality because this structure informs our beliefs and actions. I started with my own story, collected the stories of others, and discovered that an imbalance of power frequently drives human social dynamics. But then I found an even bigger story: science. I began to understand how science created and drove the daily beliefs and actions of leaders. Choosing a scientific framework was like choosing a pair of glasses. After the decision is made (which isn't conscious in the first place), we get so accustomed to wearing the glasses that we forget we have them on. What are the latest frames today to view reality? How would wearing these lenses change how we lead, live, and love?

Researchers who studied open systems were pioneers in organizational development, because these system characteristics are the same features of a complex adaptive system, while closed systems resemble the traditional hierarchical business model. A complex adaptive system (CAS) has a densely connected web of interacting agents, each operating from its own schema or local knowledge. Order and structure emerge from the group. In this framework, the CEO does not control the actions of the independent agents.

Frequently, very small changes can have large effects in this dynamic environment where relationships are so intertwined. Norms are constructed by the group in an effort to provide structure and not imposed from above. Leaders believe that people are important and relationships are absolutely vital to the smooth flow of information and energy within the system (Begun et al., 2003). People understand that while their individual roles may be different, they are all equally as vital to the life of the hospital. Staff will tell you that their managers demonstrate a great deal of caring.

These organizations feel alive with energy born of a common goal: *patient-centric care*. Attention and investment is dedicated in the form of resources for education to team building, accountability, communication, and collegial relationships. Peers keep each other in check and hostile behaviors never make it off the shift or the unit, because people understand that a healthy workplace is everyone's responsibility. For example, one small hospital needed to save a million dollars. The CEO held several emergency meetings with staff and asked, "How can we do this?" Within a week, dozens of employees decreased their FTEs, took unplanned vacation time, created job-sharing opportunities, applied for early retirement, and identified cost savings from the bedside to the boardroom. There was a "we're all in this together" feeling that permeated the entire organization. Engagement, power, creativity, and spontaneity energized the entire institution. These savings could have never been imposed from the top without resentment and anger.

When authority is diffused, responsibility becomes shared. It is imperative to use management practices aligned with the most current science.

Old vs. new management practices

OLD	NEW
Newtonian physics	Quantum physics
Hierarchy	Tribe/Team
Structure	Flow
Fear of losing control	Trusting the process
Reductionism	Holism
Linear relationships	Nonlinear relationships
Closed system	Open system
Command and control	Invite and explore
Predictable	Non-predictable
Authoritarian leadership	Authentic, resonant leadership

In contrast, the traditional hierarchical business model with the CEO at the top who can control the outcomes at the point of care has resulted in multiple directives that have had little impact on frontline behavior. Staff fondly refer to these initiatives as the "flavor of the month." This type of system functions like a machine and is based on outdated Newtonian physics principles of cause and effect—like a clock. Through this lens, acquisitions, mergers, consolidating, increasing volume, and laying off staff are all examples of actions leaders would take in order to improve the system.

Leaders in these organizations believe they can actually empower and engage staff (one hospital even had a pep rally). If you are operating in a hierarchy, then everyone knows the pecking order and understands that some people are simply more valuable because of their position. The social animal in us defends and protects our status. Horizontal hostility in this type of environment is viewed as an inconsequential Human Resources problem. Because of the corporate culture where each individual is watching out for his or her own status in order to be assured power in the hierarchy, people with higher status can get away with hostile behaviors. Exceptions to the rule create distrust, disrespect, and encourage employees to watch their backs instead of the patient.

Leaders must be aware of the conceptual model within which they are working: the glasses from which they look at their workplace every day. Each model carries with it a set of beliefs that drive our decisions. Being open to feedback is key to understanding and changing our mental models.

For the Love of Nursing

> *What we need is what the ancient Israelites called* hochma ... *the capacity to see, to feel, and then to act as if the future depended on you. Believe me, it does.*
>
> —*Bill Moyer*

In the end, it comes down to respect. According to the American Heritage Dictionary, the etymology of the word "respect" is from Middle English, *regard,* from Old French, from Latin, *respectus,* from past participle of *"respicere: to look back at, regard, consider."*

Now, I want to go back to the hospital and find Skye. I have something to say ...

We are not looking. If we could only take the time to be with and listen to each other, horizontal hostility could not exist. If we looked with intention into each other's eyes, we would see the two things we so desperately need to heal: each other's pain, and our own reflection.

We need each other. Nursing is difficult work. Building a new culture starts with rebuilding our relationships—one at a time. At this very moment, each of us knows the name of the person who *"doesn't respect me/doesn't like me/won't sit next to me/is putting me down."* And we know who we feel the same way about. Any hesitance to hold the crucial conversations necessary to heal these relationships must be immediately addressed, whether the relationships are with superiors, peers, or subordinates. Our voice—*your* voice—is the power that will liberate nursing from fear and oppression. And when that happens, all of humanity will reap the reward.

In the end, the nursing revolution we so desperately need in order to eliminate horizontal hostility will come from the deep and profound respect, compassion, and admiration we have for ourselves and each other. We just need to stop being afraid. Nelson Mandela had 27 years to think about this as he sat in prison: Why is there so much fear? For his inaugural address, he chose this quote:

> *Our deepest fear is not that we are inadequate. Our deepest fear is that we are powerful beyond measure. It is our light, not our darkness, that most frightens us. We ask ourselves, 'Who am I to be brilliant, gorgeous, talented, fabulous?' Actually, who are you not to be? … There is nothing enlightened about shrinking so that other people won't feel insecure around you. We are all meant to shine, as children do. We were born to make manifest the glory of God that is within us. It's not just in some of us; it's in everyone. And as we let our own light shine, we unconsciously give other people permission to do the same. As we are liberated from our own fear, our presence automatically liberates others.*

> — *Marianne Williamson,* A Return to Love

What is required for the general public to understand the vital role that nurses play in society? First, we must validate each other, and acknowledge our own worth. Then, each and every one of us must start sharing the stories of how our autonomous knowledge, skilled experience and compassionate bonds that we form with our patients save lives.

Nursing will not be recognized for its pivotal role in healing humanity until we tell **all** of our stories. The stories of discord that began this research are only the beginning, and represent the shadow side of our profession. But, as a wise man once said, *"Never be afraid to look into the shadows, because when you look at the shadows you will also see the light."*

Now that the shame surrounding our pain has been addressed, we are called to an even higher level: to share the magnificent healing work that nurses do every single day. These are the stories of how nurses have saved patients' lives, how educators inspired a new, highly confident generation of nurses and cutting-edge research, or of public health nurses improving the health of communities.

The time has come for nursing to "let our own light shine."

Epilogue

It seems only right that this journey that began with a story should end with one as well. Many years ago, I heard a metaphor that holds the essence of nursing's collective dilemma.

One day a nurse was walking by a river and she saw a person calling for help in the water. Immediately she waded in and pulled her out and bandaged the leg of the bleeding woman. But no sooner had she finished attending to her needs than she heard another person calling for help, then another.

She called for her friends and more nurses came to the rescue, frantically pulling injured people out of the turbulent waters. Not only did the numbers of victims increase, but the severity of their wounds did as well; so she called for the doctors. Day in and out for weeks the nurses and physicians kept saving the lives of the river wounded. Weeks turned into months, years turned into decades, and everyone was utterly exhausted.

And then one day without any warning, a single nurse stood up and started walking away from the river. Suddenly, like a swarm of swallows, thousands of nurses stood up and followed her as she walked away from the river of illness and disease. "Where are you going? You can't leave!" shouted a doctor, desperate and panicked.

Just then, the very last nurse turned back to him and shouted, "We're going to see who's throwing these people down the river."

It is time to leave the river; time to stop protecting our individual fiefdoms of professionalism and gather like moths to the flame around the value that nursing brings to our society. This coming together of like minds begins by supporting and nurturing the people we work with every day. Healing our world begins by caring for ourselves and each other with the same loving devotion that we administer to our patients.

This is our Crimean War. But because the battlefield is all around us, it is difficult to perceive exactly what we are fighting, and so, many of us are constantly drawn down to the river. If three million nurses stopped drinking bottled water or eating fast food, or demanded nurses in every school, or asked that the FDA address the use of hormones, antibiotics, and pesticides in our food supply, the number of sick people in our river of illness would decrease exponentially. This is how we can leave the paradigm of disease—and take our patients with us.

We have both an opportunity and an ethical obligation to come together in an unprecedented way to restore the health of our nation. Every individual action will either bring us closer, or further, from this goal. To that end, I hope this book has served you well.

For the love of nursing,

Kathleen

A p p e n d i x   A

Civility Assessment

One day I was presenting at a conference and met John Nelson, a statistician who has worked frequently with Jean Watson. He asked me to send him a copy of my book. A few weeks later I received an elaborate diagram in my email inbox—only a statistician could take your life's work, spin it through a mental centrifuge, and succinctly reduce the book to the one page diagram you'll see at the end of this appendix.

Dr. Nelson also wanted to test my theories, and so we collaborated with AnnMarie Papa and surveyed over 300 nurses to discover if my hypothesis were correct. The results and interpretation of that survey follow.

Civility Assessment Study

Abstract: *Testing a Theoretically Based Civility Assessment Tool and Model*
Author: *John Nelson, PhD, MS, RN*
Investigators of study: *AnnMarie Papa, Kathleen Bartholomew, John Nelson*

Background: According to the theories proposed in Bartholomew's book, the outcomes of a civil work environment is comprised of 14 dimensions: 1) staff reporting being able to act autonomously in their professional role, 2) immediate supervisor support, 3) peer support, 4) voicing concern, 5) profession is valued, 6) physicians share credit for patient care, 7) conflict management, 8) preceptor efficiency, 9) ideas from new staff welcome (no assumptions), 10) clinical learning environment, 11) relationships with physicians, 12) relationships with nurses, 13) relationship with coworkers, and 14) managerial support. Combined, positive outcomes in each one of these dimensions result in a community that embraces civility and makes civility felt by every member in the community.

Civility, according to Bartholomew, must begin in formal education. Dimensions of formal education that serve as predictors of civility include the educator(s) teaching the importance of respect of manager to staff, mentoring new staff, and educators who led by example. Professionals who are educated about and witness operationally the dimensions of civility are more likely to understand, embrace, and pursue civility within subsequent communities they belong to. Outcomes of civility, according to Bartholomew, include decreased burnout on the job and greater satisfaction with workload.

Aims: Aim one was to test the 14 dimensions of civility using factor analysis. Aim two was to examine if formal education experience was a predictor of civility. Aim three was to test if outcomes of civility include decreased workload and increased satisfaction with workload. Aim four was to describe perception of civility among nurse demographics.

Method: This descriptive study utilized a cross-sectional sample of staff nurses employed in acute care in the Northeastern portion of the United States of America. After ethics committee approval, an email was sent to all potential respondents using a secure Internet link. Respondents were able to "save and return" to their survey regarding civility as often as they'd like. Exploratory factor analysis procedures were employed to examine the factor structure of the proposed 14 dimensions of civility. Hierarchical regression was proposed be used to examine predictors of civility.

Findings: There were 154 of 388 nurses who responded (a 40% response rate). Of the 154 returned, there were 148 surveys complete and used for analysis. Seven units from three different service lines participated. Among respondents, there were 135 licensed staff and 19 unlicensed. The most common role was Clinical Nurse I and II (n = 66 and 25, respectively). There were 41 total items that loaded in the final factor analysis. The Kaiser-Meyer-Olkin (KMO) was .86 and the Bartlett's Test of

Sphericity was significant (p = .000), indicating the sample was adequate to conduct a PCA. The cutoff for entry into the PCA was .30. Scree Plot revealed 9 dimensions with eigenvalues greater than 1.0. Combined, the 14 subscales explained 74% of the variance of civility. Cronbach's alpha for all subscales were above .70. The sample was not large enough to conduct hierarchical regression, so Pearson's correlations were used to examine how civility related to predictors and outcomes. All three predictors have a positive relationship to civility, including educator led by example (r = .30, p = .001), educator taught importance of respect by managers to staff (r = .29, p = .001), and educator taught how to nurture new staff (r = .32, p = < .001). The proposed outcomes of burnout had a negative relationship with burnout (r = 0.215, p = .013) and positive relationship with satisfaction with workload (r = .52, p = < .001). No differences were found when comparing service lines in relationship to perception of civility.

Conclusion/Implications: The Civility Assessment tested in this study provides an initial valid instrument to research civility. In addition, the proposed model, based on Bartholomew's theory of civility, was validated as true for the sample of respondents in this setting. Additional testing of the Civility Assessment and associated model in additional settings is warranted. Interventions targeted to increasing civility should be tested to identify what strategies enhance civility thus enhance satisfaction with concurrent decreased burnout for clinical care staff. Finally, the finding that the academic setting prior to clinical practice impacts perception of civility should be studied further.

Visual Map: Refer to the visual map for an overview of roles and responsibilities related to assessing and addressing lateral (horizontal) hostility in the nursing environment.

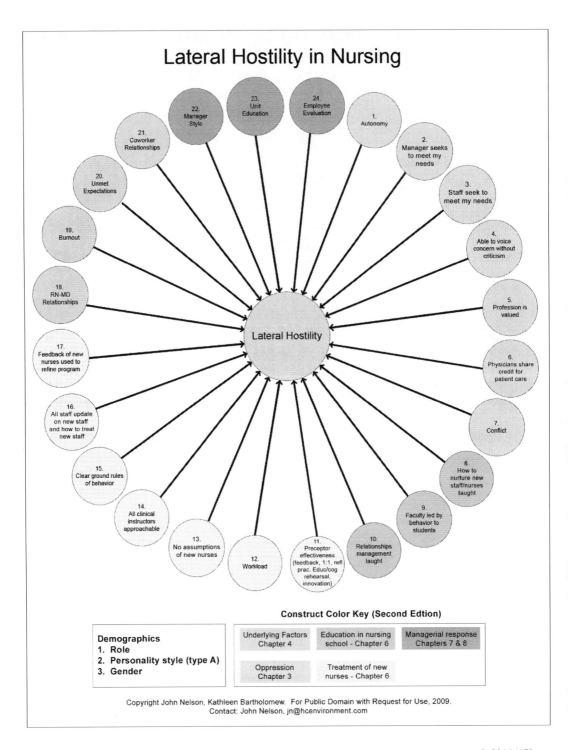

A p p e n d i x   B

Bibliography

Adams, A. (1997). *Bullying at Work: How to Confront and Overcome It.* London: Virago Press.

Aiken, L., et al. (2001). Nurses' reports on hospital care in five countries. *Health Affairs* 20(3): 43–53.

Aiken, L., et al. (2002). Hospital nurse staffing and patient mortality, nurse burnout, and job dissatisfaction. *Journal of the American Medical Association* 288: 1987–1993.

Aiken, L., et al. (2010). Implications of the California nurse staffing mandate for other states. *Health Services Research* 45(4): 904–921.

Almost, J., Laschinger, H., & Tuer-Hodes, D. (2003). Workplace empowerment and Magnet hospital characteristics. *Journal of Nursing Administration* 33: 410–422.

American Association of Colleges of Nursing. Nursing Shortage Fact Sheet. *www.aacn.nche.edu/Media/shortageresource.htm.*

Amos, M., Hu, H., & Herrick, C. (2005). The impact of team building on communication and job satisfaction of nursing staff. *Journal for Nurses in Staff Development* 21(1).

Anderson, C., & Stamper, M. (2001). Workplace violence. *RN* 64(2): 71–74.

Araujo, S., & Sofield, L. (1999). Verbal Abuse. *www.home.comcast.net/~laura08723/article2.htm.*

Ariely, D. (2010). *Predictably Irrational.* New York: Harper Perennial.

Arle, L. (2004). Horizontal Caring in Nursing and a Narrative Community Experience. Unpublished thesis for Masters in Nursing. Washington State University, Washington.

Aronson, E., Wilson T.D., & Akert, R.M. (2005). *Social Psychology*, 7th ed. Upper Saddle River, NJ: Pearson Education, Inc.

Auerbach, D., et al. (2013). The nursing workforce in an era of healthcare reform. *New England Journal of Medicine* 368: 1470–1472.

Baggs, J., et al. (1999). Association between nurse-physician collaboration and patient outcomes in three intensive care units. *Critical Care Medicine* 27(9): 1998–1999.

Bartholomew, K., & Byrum, S. (2010). Harm is not an option. *The OR Connection, Medline.*

Bartholomew, K. (2004). *Speak Your Truth: Proven Strategies for Effective Nurse-Physician Communication.* Marblehead, MA: HCPro.

Bartholomew, K. (2010). A failure to rescue ourselves. *American Journal of Nursing.* 110(11).

Bartholomew, K. (2012). Survey to members of the Student Nurses Association.

Bartholomew, K. (2013). Hospital Impact Blog. *www.hospitalimpact.org/index.php/2013/ 04/24/hospitals_do_you_have_what_it_takes_to_a.*

Begun, J., Zimmerman B., & Dooley, K. (2003). Health care organizations as complex adaptive systems. In S. M. Mick & M. Wyttenbach (eds.), *Advances in Health Care Organization Theory* (pp. 253–288).San Francisco: Jossey-Bass.

Blegen, M. (1993). Nurses' job satisfaction: A meta-analysis of related variables. *Nursing Research* 42(1): 36–41.

Boughn, S. (1992). Nursing students rank high in autonomy at the exit level. *Journal of Nursing Education* 31(2): 58–64.

Braun, K., et al. (1991). Verbal abuse of nurses and non-nurses. *Nursing Management* 22(30): 72–76.

Brooks, D. (2011). *The Social Animal: The Hidden Sources of Love, Character, and Achievement.* New York: Random House.

Brownlee, S. (2007). *Overtreated: Why Too Much Medicine Is Making Us Sicker and Poorer.* New York: Bloomsbury.

Buback, D. (2004). Home study program: Assertiveness training to prevent verbal abuse in the OR. *AORN Journal* 79(1): 148–164.

Bully Busting Bill 168. (2009). *www.juiceinc.com/articles/show/the-bully-busting-bill-ontarios-bill-168*, Ontario, Canada.

Bunk, J., & Magley, V. (2013). The role of appraisals and emotions in understanding experiences of workplace incivility. *Journal of Occupational Health Psychology* 18(1): 87–105.

Buresh, B., & Gordon S. (2003). *From Silence to Voice: What Nurses Know and Must Communicate to the Public*. Ithaca, NY: Cornell University Press.

Cacioppo, J., et al. (2008). Loneliness: The structure and spread of loneliness in a large social network. www.*psychology.uchicago.edu/people/faculty/cacioppo/jtcreprints/cfc09.pdf*.

Canadian Nurses Association. (2008). *Code of Ethics*. Ottawa, ON.

Cartwright, S., & Cooper, C. (1993). The psychological impact of merger and acquisition on the individual: A study of building society managers. *Human Relations* 46(3): 327–348.

Cathcart, D., et al. (2004). Span of control matters. *Journal of Nursing Administration* 34(9): 395–399.

Center for American Nurses. (2007). Position statement on work environment: Restructuring and redesign of nurses' work environments. *Nebraska Nurse*. 40(4): 20–21.

Ceravolo, D. J., et al. (2012). Strengthening communication to overcome lateral violence. *Journal of Nursing Management* 20: 599–606.

Chambliss, D. (1996). *Beyond Caring: Hospitals, Nurses, and the Social Organization of Ethics*. Chicago, IL: University of Chicago Press.

Charney, W. (2011). *Epidemic of Medical Errors and Hospital-Acquired Infections: A Systemic Approach*. Boca Raton, FL: CRC Press.

Cho, S.H., et al. (2012). Turnover of new graduate nurses in their first job using survival analysis. *Journal of Nursing Scholarship* 44(1): 63–70.

Clark, C. (2013). *Creating and Sustaining Civility in Nursing Education*. Indianapolis, IN: Sigma Theta Tau International.

Clipper, B. (2012). *The Nurse Manager's Guide to an Intergenerational Workforce*. Indianapolis: Sigma Theta Tau International.

Clippinger, J.H. (2007). *A Crowd of One: The Future of Individual Identity*. New York: Public Affairs.

Cook, J., et al. (2001). Exploring the impact of physician verbal abuse on perioperative nurses. *AORN Journal* 74(3): 317–330.

Cook, T., et al. (2003). Beginning students' definitions of nursing: an inductive framework of professional identity. *Journal of Nurse Educators* 42(7): 311–317.

Copeland, W. (2013). Bullying's lifelong damage. *The Week*, March 15, 2013.

Cornell, A.W. (2013). *Focusing in Clinical Practice: The Essence of Change.* New York, NY: Norton and Co.

Cortina, L., et al. (2001). Incivility in the workplace: Incidence and impact. *Journal of Occupational Health Psychology* 6(1): 64–80.

Cox, H. (1991). Verbal abuse nationwide, part II: Impact and modifications. *Nursing Management* 22(3): 66–69.

Cox, K. (2003). The effects of intrapersonal, intragroup, and intergroup conflict on team performance effectiveness and work satisfaction. *Nursing Administration Quarterly* 27(2).

Croft, R.K., & Cash, P.A. (2012). Deconstructing contributing factors to bullying and lateral violence in nursing using a postcolonial feminist lens. *Contemporary Nurse* 42(2): 226–242.

Daiski, I. (2004). Changing nurses' disempowering relationship patterns. *Journal of Advanced Nursing* 48(1): 43–50.

Dargon, M. (1999). Disrupting Oppression Theory. Unpublished thesis for Masters in Nursing. University of Tasmania, Launceston, Australia.

Davey, L. (2002). Nurses eating nurses: The caring profession which fails to nurture its own. *Contemporary Nurse* 13(2–3): 192–197.

David, B. (2000). Nursing's gender politics: Reformulating the footnotes. *Advances in Nursing Science* 23(1): 83–93.

DeMarco, R., Roberts, S., & Chandler, G. (2005). The use of a writing group to enhance voice and connection among staff nurses. *Journal for Nurses in Staff Development* 21(3): 85–90.

Donadio, G. (2012). *Changing Behavior.* Boston: SoulWork Press.

Doran, D., et al. (2004). Impact of the manager's span of control on leadership and performance. Canadian Health Services Research Foundation. *www.chsrf.ca.*

Dunn, H. (2003). Horizontal violence among nurses in the operating room. *AORN Journal* 78(6).

Ebright, P., et al. (2003). Understanding the complexity of registered nurse work in acute care settings. *Journal of Nursing Administration* 33(12).

Edmondson, A. (2012). Teamwork on the fly. *Harvard Business Review*, April, 2012.

Emdad, R., et al. (2012). The impact of bystanding to workplace bullying on symptoms of depression among women and men in industry in Sweden: An empirical and theoretical longitudinal study. *International Archives of Occupational & Environmental Health*, doi: 10.1007/s00420-012-0813-1.

Emergency Nurses Association. (2011). Emergency department violence surveillance study 16. Accessed September 27, 2012, *www.ena.org/IENR/Documents/NAEDVSReportNovember2011.pdf.*

Emerick, T., & Lewis, A. (2013). *Cracking Health Costs*, Fourteenth Edition. Hoboken: Wiley.

Erickson, R., & Grove, W. (2007). Why emotions matter: Age, agitation, and burnout among registered nurses. *The Online Journal of Issues in Nursing*. Available at *http://tinyurl.com/mutfn6v.*

Falk-Rafael, A. (1996). Power and caring: A dialectic in nursing. *Advances in Nursing Science* 19(1): 3–17.

Farrell, G. (1997). Aggression in clinical settings: Nurses' views. *Journal of Advanced Nursing* 25: 501–508.

Farrell, G. (1999). Aggression in clinical settings: Nurses' views—A follow-up study. *Journal of Advanced Nursing* 29(3): 532–541.

Farrell, G. (2001). From tall poppies to squashed weeds: Why don't nurses pull together more? *Journal of Advanced Nursing* 35(1): 26–33.

Farrell, G. (2005). Unpublished SWAN study presented at the Violence in the Workplace conference. Tualatin, OR. Sponsored by the Oregon Chapter of the American Psychiatric Nurses Association.

Felps, W., Mitchell, T.R., & Byington, E. (2006). How, when, and why bad apples spoil the barrel. *Research in Organizational Behavior* 27: 175–222.

Freire, P. (1990). *Pedagogy of the Oppressed*. New York: Continuum International Publishing Group.

Freshwater, D. (2000). Crosscurrents: Against cultural narration in nursing. *Journal of Advanced Nursing* 32(2).

Gates, D., Gillespie, G., & Succop, P. (2011). Violence against nurses and its impact on stress and productivity. *Nursing Economic$* 29(2).

Geiger-Brown J., et al. (2012). Sleep, sleepiness, fatigue, and performance of 12-hour shift nurses. *Chronobiology International* 29(2): 211–219.

Gendlin, E. (2007). Focusing: The body speaks from the inside, Talk given at the 18th Annual International Trauma Conference. *www.focusing.org/gendlin/docs/gol_2235.html*

Gilmour, D., & Hamlin, L. (2003). Bullying and harassment in perioperative settings. *British Journal of Perioperative Nursing* 13(2): 79–85.

Glass, N. (2003). Studying women nurse academics: Exposing workplace violence in Australia: Part 2. *Contemporary Nurse* 14: 187–195.

Glass, N. (2007). Investigating women nurse academics' experiences in universities: The importance of hope, optimism, and career resilience for workplace satisfaction. In M.H. Oermann & K. T. Heinrich (Eds.), *Annual Review of Nursing Education* (5: pp. 111–136). New York: Springer.

Goldenberg, D., & Waddell, J. (1990). Occupational stress and coping strategies among female baccalaureate nursing faculty. *Journal of Advanced Nursing* 15(5): 531–543.

Gordon, S. (2005). *Nursing Against the Odds: How Healthcare Cost-Cutting, Media Stereotypes, and Medical Hubris Undermine Nurses and Patient Care* (The Culture and Politics of Healthcare Work). Ithaca, NY: ILR Press.

Griffin, M. (2004). Teaching cognitive rehearsal as a shield for lateral violence: An Intervention for newly licensed nurses. *The Journal of Continuing Education in Nursing* 35(6).

Haidt, J. (2012). *The Righteous Mind: Why Good People Are Divided by Politics and Religion*. New York: Pantheon Books.

Harris, K.J., et al. (2013). An investigation of abusive supervision, vicarious supervision, and their joint impacts. *Journal of Social Psychology* 153(1): 38–50.

Hart, A. (1993). *The Crazy-Making Workplace*. Ann Arbor, MI: Servant Publications.

Health Quality Council of Alberta. (2013). Managing Disruptive Behavior in the Healthcare Workplace. *Provincial Framework* Canada. *www.hqca.ca/index.php?id–281.*

Heinrich, K.T. (2007). Joy-stealing games: 10 mean games faculty play and how to stop the gaming. *Nurse Educator* 32(1): 34–38.

Heinrich, K.T. (2006). Joy-stealing games. Reflections on nursing leadership. Retrieved April 18, 2009, from *http://nursingsociety.org/RNL/2Q_2006/features/feature5.html.*

Hershcovis, M.S. (2011). Incivility, social undermining, bullying...Oh my!: A call to reconcile constructs within the workplace aggression research. *Journal of Organizational Behavior* 32: 499–519.

Hillhouse, J., & Adler, C. (1997). Investigating stress effect patterns in hospital staff nurses: Results of a cluster analysis. *Social Science and Medicine* 45(12): 1781–1788.

Hilton, P., Kottke, J., & Pfahler, D. (1994). Verbal abuse in nursing: How serious is it? *Nursing Management* 25(5): 90.

Hutchinson, M., et al. (2006). Workplace bullying in nursing: Towards a more critical organisational perspective. *Nursing Inquiry* 13(2): 118–126.

Hutchinson, M., et al. (2010). A typology of bullying behaviours: The experiences of Australian nurses. *Journal of Clinical Nursing* 19: 2319–2328.

Hutton, S. & Gates, D. (2008). Workplace incivility and productivity losses among direct care staff. *AAOHN Journal* 56(4): 168–175.

Institute of Medicine (2007). *Preventing Medication Errors.* Washington, D.C.: The National Acadamies Press.

Jack, D.C. (1993). *Silencing the Self: Women and Depression.* New York: William Morrow.

Jackson, D., Firtko, A., & Edenborough, M. (2007). Personal resilience as a strategy for surviving and thriving in the face of workplace adversity: A literature review. *Journal of Advanced Nursing* 60(1): 1–9.

James, J.T. (2013). A new, evidence-based estimate of patient harms associated with hospital care. *Journal of Patient Safety* 9(3): 122–128.

Kanter, R. (1979). Power failure in management circuits. *Harvard Business Review* 57(4): 65–75.

Katz, D., & Kahn, R. (1978). *The Social Psychology of Organizations*, 2nd edition. New York: Wiley.

Keuter, K., et al. (2000). Nurses' job satisfaction and organizational climate in a dynamic work environment. *Applied Nursing Research* 13(1): 46–49.

Kramer, M. (1974). *Reality Shock: Why Nurses Leave Nursing.* St. Louis, MO: The C.V. Mosby Company.

Krichbaum, K., et al. (2007). Complexity compression: Nurses under fire. *Nursing Forum* 42(2).

Kupperschmidt, B. (2008). Conflicts at work? Try carefronting. *Journal of Christian Nursing*, 25(1): 10–17. *www.medscape.com/viewarticle/774256_3*.

Larson, E. (1999). The impact of physician-nurse interaction on patient care. *Holistic Nursing Practice* 13(2): 38–47.

Laschinger, H.K., et al. (2013). Workplace incivility and new graduate nurses' mental health: the protective role of resiliency. *Journal of Nursing Administration*. 43(7–8): 415–421.

Leppa, C. (1996). Nurse relationships and work group disruption. *Journal of Nursing Administration* 26(10): 23–27.

Logan, D., King, J., & Fischer-Wright, H. (2008). *Tribal Leadership: Leveraging Groups to Build a Thriving Organization*. New York: HarperBusiness.

Lyndon, A. et al. (2011). Predicting likelihood of speaking up in labor and delivery. *Journal of Obstetric, Gynecologic, & Neonatal Nursing* 40: S117–S118.

Magee, J., & Galinsky, A. (2008). Social hierarchy: The self-reinforcing nature of power and status. *The Academy of Management Annals* 2(1): 351–398.

Manderino, M., & Berkey, N. (1997). Verbal abuse of staff nurses by physicians. *Journal of Professional Nursing* 13(1): 48–55.

Mantzoukas, S., & Jasper, M. (2004). Reflective practice and daily ward reality: A covert power game. *Journal of Clinical Nursing* 13(8): 925–933.

Marche, S. (2012). Is Facebook making us lonely? *Atlantic Monthly*, May 2012.

Mark, B., et al. (2013). California's minimum nurse staffing legislation: Results from a natural experiment. *Health Services Research*. 48(2pt1): 435–454. doi:10.1111/j.1475-6773.2012.01465.x

Marks, M., & Mirvis, P. (1992). Rebuilding after the merger: Dealing with survivor sickness. *Organizational Dynamics* 21(2): 18–33.

Martin, S., & Klein, A. (2013). The presumption of mutual influence in occurrences of workplace bullying: Time for change. *Journal of Aggression, Conflict and Peace Research* 5(3): 147–155.

Matthews, S., et al. (2006). Staff nurse empowerment in line and staff organizational structures for chief nurse executives. *Journal of Nursing Administration* 36(11): 526–533.

May, D., & Grubbs, L. (2002). The extent, nature, and precipitating factors of nurse assault among three groups of registered nurses in a regional medical center. *Journal of Emergency Nursing* 28(3): 191.

Mayhew, C., et al. (2004). Measuring the extent of impact from occupational violence and bullying on traumatized workers. *Employee Responsibilities and Rights Journal* 16: 117–134.

McCann, C., et al. Resilience in the health professions: A review of recent literature. *International Journal of Wellbeing*, 3(1), 60–81. doi:10.5502/ijw.v3il.4

McDonough, W. (2002). Institute of Noetic Sciences Conference. Palm Springs, CA.

McKenna, B., et al. (2003). Horizontal violence: Experiences of registered nurses in their first year of practice. *Journal of Advanced Nursing* 42(1): 90–96.

McMillan, I. (1995). Losing Control. *Nursing Times* 91(15): 40–43.

Mick, S. M., & Wyttenbach, M. (eds.), (2003). *Advances in Health Care Organization Theory.* (pp. 253–288). San Francisco: Jossey-Bass.

Moses Cone Health System. New Graduates: Graduate Advancement Program. *www.mosescone.com/body.cfm?id–540.*

Namie, G., & Namie, R. (2000). *The Bully at Work: What You Can Do to Stop the Hurt and Reclaim Your Dignity on the Job.* Naperville, IL: Sourcebooks, Inc.

Nance, J. (2009). *Why Hospitals Should Fly.* Second River Healthcare, Bozeman, MT.

National Center for Victims of Crime (2014). 2014 National Crime Victims' Rights Week Resource Guide. *http://ovc.ncjrs.gov/ncvrw2014/index.html.*

Neily, J., et al. (2010). Association between implementation of a medical team training program and surgical mortality *JAMA.* 304(15): 1693–1700. doi: 10.1001/jama.2010.1506.

Newman, M. (2008). *Transforming Presence: The Difference Nursing Makes.* Philadelphia: F.A. Davis.

O'Hare, M., & O'Hare, J. (2004). Don't perpetuate horizontal violence. *Nursing Spectrum.*

Patterson, K., et al. (2002). *Crucial Conversation: Tools for Talking When Stakes are High.* New York: McGraw-Hill Trade.

Pentland, A. (2012). The new science of building great teams. *Harvard Business Review.* April 2012.

Perissinotto, C., Stijacici Cenzer, I., & Covinsky, K. (2012). Loneliness in older persons: A predictor of functional decline and death. *Archives of Internal Medicine* 172(14): 1078–1083.

Pink, D. (2010). *Drive*. New York: Riverhead Books.

Porath, C., & Erez, A. (2007). Does rudeness really matter? The effects of rudeness on task performance and helpfulness. *Academy of Management Journal* 50(5): 1181–1197.

Porath, C., & Pearson, C. (2009). *The Cost of Bad Behavior: How Incivility Is Damaging Your Business and What to Do About It*. London: Penguin Books.

Porter O'Grady, T. (2005). *Shared Governance: How to Create and Sustain a Culture of Nurse Empowerment*. Marblehead, MA: HCPro.

Purpora, C. (2010). *Horizontal Violence Among Hospital Staff Nurses and the Quality and Safety of Patient Care*. PhD dissertation, Univ. of CA, San Francisco (Publication No. AAT 3426213).

Purpora, C., Blegen, M., & Stotts, N. (2012). Horizontal violence among hospital staff nurses related to oppressed self or oppressed group. *Journal of Professional Nursing* 28(5): 306–314.

Putnam, R. (2000). *Bowling Alone: The Collapse and Revival of American Community*. New York: Simon & Schuster.

Quine, L. (1999). Workplace bullying in NHS Community Trust: Staff questionnaire survey. *British Medical Journal* 318: 228–232.

Quinn, D. (2009). *Beyond Civilization*. New York: Random House.

Randle, J. (2003). Bullying in the nursing profession. *Journal of Advanced Nursing* 43(4): 395–401.

Reverby, S. (1987). *Ordered to Care: The Dilemma of American Nursing 1850–1945*. New York: Cambridge University Press.

Roberts, S. (1983). Oppressed group behavior: Implications for nursing. *Advances in Nursing Science* 5(4): 21–30.

Robinson, E. (2013). *The Soul of the Nurse*. Santa Barbara, CA: SpannRobinson.

Rocker, C.F. (2008). Addressing nurse-to-nurse bullying to promote nurse retention. *The Online Journal of Issues in Nursing* 13(3): 1–10.

Rodwell, C. (1996). An analysis of the concept of empowerment. *Journal of Advanced Nursing* 23(2): 305–313.

Rodwell, J., & Demir, D. (2012). Psychological consequences of bullying for hospital and aged care nurses. *International Nursing Review* 59(4): 539–546.

Rosenstein, A. (2002). Nurse-physician relationships: Impact on nurse satisfaction and retention. *Advanced Journal of Nursing* 102(6): 26–34.

Rosenstein, A., & O'Daniel, M. (2008). A survey of the impact of disruptive behaviors and communication defects on patient safety. *www.mc.vanderbilt.edu/root/pdfs/nursing/ppb_article_on_disruptive.pdf.*

Rosenstein, A., & Naylor, B. (2011). Incidence and impact of disruptive physician and nurse behaviors in the emergency room. *Journal of Emergency Medicine, www.physiciandisruptivebehavior.com/admin/articles/24.pdf.*

Sado, S., & Bayer, A. (2001). Executive Summary: The Changing American Family. *Population Resource Center.*

Sapolsky, R. (1998). *Why Zebras Don't Get Ulcers: An Updated Guide to Stress, Stress-Related Diseases, and Coping.* New York: Freeman & Company.

Schoessler, M. (2005). *Narrative Community for Newly Graduated Nurses.* Self-published.

Scholtes, P. (1988). *The Team Handbook.* Madison, WI: Joiner Associates, Inc.

Scott, L., et al. (2006). Effects of critical care nurses' work hours on vigilance and patients' safety. *American Journal of Critical Care* 15(1).

Seligman, M. et al. (2005). Positive psychology progress: Empirical validation of interventions. *American Psychologist* 60(5): 410–421.

Simmons, R. (2002). *Odd Girl Out: The Hidden Culture of Aggression in Girls.* New York: Mariner Books, Houghton Mifflin.

Simons, S. (2008). Workplace bullying experienced by Massachusetts registered nurses and the relationship to intention to leave the organization. *Advances in Nursing Science.* 31(2):E48–E59.

Smith, M., Droppleman, P., & Thomas, S. (1996). Under assault: The experience of work-related anger in female registered nurses. *Nursing Forum* 31(1): 22–33.

Sofield, L., & Salmond, S. (2003). Workplace violence: A focus on verbal abuse and intent to leave the organization. *Orthopaedic Nursing* 22(4): 274–283.

Sommers, S. (2011). *Situations Matter: Understanding How Context Transforms Your World*. New York: Riverhead Books, Penguin.

Steptoe, A., et al. (2013). Social isolation, loneliness and all-cause mortality in older men and women. *Proceedings of the National Academy of Sciences*, 110(15): 5733–5734.

Sternberg, R., & Horvath, J. (1998). *Tacit Knowledge in Professional Practice*. Mahwah, NJ: Lawrence Erlbaum Associates.

Stockowski, L. (2013). The 4-generation gap in nursing. Medscape.com, *www.medscape.com/viewarticle/781752*.

Sumner, J., & Townsend-Rocchiccioli, J. (2003). Why are nurses leaving nursing? *Nursing Administration Quarterly* 27(2): 164–171.

Thomas, S. (2003). 'Horizontal hostility'—Nurses against themselves: How to resolve this threat to retention. *Journal of Advanced Nursing* 103(10).

Thomas, S. (2004). *Transforming Nurses' Stress and Anger: Steps Toward Healing*. New York: Springer Publishing Company.

Thomas, S., & Jozwiak, J. (1990). Self attitudes and behavioral characteristics of type A and B female registered nurses. *Healthcare for Women International* 11: 477–489.

Thomas, S.P., & Burk, R. (2009). Junior nursing students experience of vertical violence during clinical rotation. *Nursing Outlook*, 57: 4226–4231.

Torres, G. (1981). The nursing education administrator: Accountable, vulnerable, and oppressed. *Advances in Nursing Science* 3: 1–16.

Tucker, A., & Spear, S. (2006). Operational failures and interruptions in hospital nursing. *Health Services Research* 41(3 Pt 1): 643–662.

Ulrich, B., et al. (2010). Improving retention, confidence, and competence of new graduate nurses: Results from a 10-year longitudinal database. *Nursing Economic$* 28(6).

Upenieks, V. (2003). The interrelationship of organizational characteristics of Magnet hospitals, nursing leadership and nursing job satisfaction. *Health Care Manager* 22(2): 83–97.

Vessey, J.A., DeMarco, R., & DiFazio, R. (2011). Bullying, harassment, and horizontal violence in the nursing workforce: The state of science. *Annual Review of Nursing Research* 28: 133–157.

Viverais-Dresler, G., & Kutschke, M. (2001). RN students' ratings and opinions related to the importance of certain clinical teacher behaviors. *Journal of Continuing Education in Nursing* 32(6): 274–282.

Wagner, S. E. (2006). Staff retention: From 'satisfied' to 'engaged.' *Nursing Management* 37: 24–29.

Walrafen, N., et al. (2012). Sadly caught up in the moment: An exploration of horizontal violence. *Nursing Economic$* 30(1).

Walumbwa, F., et al. (2008). Authentic leadership: development and validation of a theory based measure. *Journal of Management*, 34: 89–126.

Weaver, K. (2013). The effects of horizontal violence and bullying on new nurse retention. *Journal for Nurses in Professional Development* 29(3): 138–142.

Weinberg, D. (2003). *Code Green: Money-Driven Hospitals and the Dismantling of Nursing*. Ithaca, NY: Cornell University Press.

Weller, J., Boyd, M., & Cumin, D. (2014). Teams, tribes and patient safety: overcoming barriers to effective teamwork in healthcare. *Postgrad Medical Journal*, doi: 10.1136/postgradmedj-2012-131168.

Wheatley, M. (2002). *Turning to One Another: Simple Conversations to Restore Hope to the Future*. San Francisco: Berrett-Koehler.

Wicks, R. (2005). *Overcoming Secondary Stress in Medical and Nursing Practice*. United Kingdom: Oxford University Press.

Witkowski-Stimpfel, A., Sloane, D., & Aiken, L. (2012). The longer the shifts for hospital nurses, the higher the levels of burnout and patient dissatisfaction. *HealthAffairs* 31(11): 2501–2509.

Zeoli, A., et al. (2014). Homicide as Infectious Disease: Using Public Health Methods to Investigate the Diffusion of Homicide. *Justice Quarterly* 31(3): 609–632.